Chinese

Japanese

Korean

French

German

Russian

Vietnamese

English

Latin

MULTI-LANGUAGE LEXICON OF ACUPUNCTURE POINT NAMES

Carole I. Binswanger, M.A., M.Ac. (U.K.)

Element Books

*Jacket and book design and production by
Kathleen Westray and Ed Sturmer.*

ISBN 0 906540 83 6

Library of Congress Catalog Card Number: 85-090368
Published by Element Books Ltd, Longmead, Shaftesbury, Dorset
Printed in Great Britain by Robert Hartnoll Limited, Bodmin, Cornwall

To mutual understanding;

a bridge across many languages

Preface

The Lexicon has been compiled in an effort to ease communication in the science of acupuncture, hopefully to aid in research, and to act as a bridge towards exchange and understanding of previously written material in the field during this period of transition in which we are moving towards a universal language.

In an effort to be on the one hand comprehensive and on the other to have a text which is simple, to facilitate the cross-reference of acupuncture material, it was decided to cross-reference only those languages with the greatest written historical material.

As this text was undertaken as a partial requirement for a Bachelor's Degree in Acupuncture by the School for Traditional Acupuncture, Oxford, England, the point system is in keeping with that employed by Prof. J. R. Worsley.

In attempting to unify the point terms of the various countries, it became clear that there were two major areas of difference with respect to the points of the Governor Vessel and Bladder meridians. In order that the points on a given line would correspond the following format was carried out: The Governor vessel is listed as having 28 points. This means that for those systems utilizing 27 points, the reader need only advance one number beginning with #7 through #27; that is, #8 will be #9, etc.

The other adaptation has been on the Bladder Meridian, in which the point at the beginning of the second Bladder line at the level of the thorasic vertebrae 3-4 is noted as point #36, and the next sequence of points advance one until point #54 at the center of the posterior knee.

The Chinese Pinyin text is in accordance with the latest name changes suggested by the Working Group on the Standardization of Acupuncture Nomenclature which, as part of the World Health Organization for the Western-Pacific Region, met in Manila December 14-20, 1982. Their determination was that, in light of the fact that the Chinese written characters make a distinction between all points, it was inappropriate to add anatomical notations to distinguish points translated in different languages with the same name. (An example would be Neck-Futu and Femur Futu.) For purposes of this Lexicon, to facilitate its use by those readers who are familiar with the anatomical reference note the following: 1. Within the numerical/numbered listing the anatomical names have been placed in brackets, 2. in the other sections where the Pinyin is represented, in looking for points previously denoted by anatomical designation, one can find the points by reference to the second word of the point name.

Certain omissions have been made. Not included are the "newer" extra or extraordinary points. As the basic tenet of this text is to cull together acupuncture points which have been represented by different names from one country to another, this has not been an issue in communication with these more recent notations.

There has also been no attempt to include the Auricular points within this volume, for the points denoted by the Chinese and P.F.M. Nogier in many instances rely on different mappings of the ear, and on different philosophical premises, rather than as a result of terminological disparity.

Spanish speaking countries have recently incorporated the current Chinese Pinyin terms for acupuncture points, so that no separate listing is included here.

French acupuncturists were among the first non-orientals to investigate this science, and a number of masters working independently of each other produced texts utilizing different translations of the Chinese characters. In the interest of making this first Lexicon most concise, the work of Soulie de Morant, as an early scholar, has been the one incorporated in the body of the text. To be in synchrony with the rest of the text the translations of the Chinese points by Soulie de Morant are included, adapting the numbering system in accordance with the Chinese characters they represent. Acknowledgement, meanwhile, is also made to the major contributions of de la Fuye, Chamfrault, Lavier, and the newer contributions of Van Nghi, Requena, Shatz, Laire, Colin, and Auteroche.

The number of languages presented for the "eight extra meridians" varies. The Governing and Conception meridian points have been translated in most languages, and within this text have been included with the major meridians. Although the extra six meridians are composed of points already listed on the major meridians there is a great deal of variation as to the number and particularity of points included in each instance. All those available to the author have been incorporated here.

Perhaps the greatest challenge arises in translating the ancient characters into English. Since the author recognizes the extreme difficulty, and maybe even arrogance, of a person not only many centuries removed but in addition not even of Chinese tongue making decisions as to the authenticity of a translation, there has been an attempt to offset this by employing a number of translations. Though recognizing there still will be many flaws, it was felt the value readers might gain in appreciation of the poetic as well as the therapeutic implications of the names of the points warranted this risk.

Any such work is possible only through the cooperation and help from people around the world, and the author would like to give special thanks to John Moore, Dr. K.C. Ho, Wataru Ohashi, Collette Guinebert, Linda Zuckerman, and Dr. Yves Requena, for the time given from their very busy schedules and for their assistance which has ensured the breadth of this project.

Contents

Scheme

I	Heart	HT
II	Small Intestine	SI
III	Bladder	BL
IV	Kidney	KI
V	Circulation-Sex	CS
VI	Three Heater	TH
VII	Gall Bladder	GB
VIII	Liver	LV
IX	Lung	LU
X	Large Intestine	LI
XI	Stomach	ST
XII	Spleen	SP
XIII	Conception Vessel	CV
XIV	Governor Vessel	GV

NUMBERED

SYSTEM

Heart Meridian

N	Cc	P	W	J	Kc	K
I.1	极泉	Jiquán	Chichuan	Kyokusen	극 천	Geug-Cheon
I.2	青灵	Qīnglíng	Chingling	Seirei	청 령	Cheong-Lyeong
I.3	少海	Shàohǎi	Shaohai	Shōkai	소 해	Eum-So-Hae
I.4	灵道	Língdào	Lingtao	Reidō	영 도	Yeong-Do
I.5	通里	Tōnglǐ	Tungli	Tsūri	통 리	Tong-Ri
I.6	阴郄	Yīnxì	Yinhsi	Ingeki	음 극	Eum-Geug
I.7	神门	Shénmén	Shenmen	Shinmon	신 문	Sin-Mun
I.8	少府	Shàofǔ	Shaofu	Shōfu	소 부	So-Bu
I.9	少冲	Shàochōng	Shaochung	Shōshō	소 충	So-Chung

N = Numbered system · Cc = Han Chinese characters · P = Pinyin Chinese
W = Wade-Giles Chinese · J = Japanese · Kc = Korean characters · K = Korean

F	G	R	V	L
Tsi-Ts'iuann	Höchste Quelle	Цзи-цюань	Cuc-tuyën	Fons culminis
Tsring-Ling	Jung-Seele	Цин-лин	Thanh-linh	Fons caeruleus
Chao-Rae	Geringes Meer	Шао-хай	Thiëu-hāi	Mare minus
Ling-Tao	Geisterweg	Лин-дао	Linh-dao	Foramen responsivum
Trong-Li	Verbindung mit dem Inneren	Тун-ли	Thong-ly	Vicus comunicans
Inn-Tsri	Yin-Grenze	Инь-си	Âm-ky	Rimicum yin minoris
Chenn-Menn	Göttliches Tor	Шэнь-мэнь	Thàn-mōn	Impedimentale laetitiae
Chao-Fou	Geringer Bezirk	Шао-фу	Thièu-phū	Aula minor
Chao-Tsrong	Geringer Angriffspunkt	Шао-чун	Thiēu-xung	Impedimentale minus

F = French · G = German · R = Russian
V = Vietnamese · L = Latin

Small Intestine Meridian

N	Cc	P	W	J	Kc	K
II.1	少泽	Shaozé	Shaotse	Shōtaku	소 택	So-Taeg
II.2	前谷	Qiángŭ	Chienku	Zenkoku	전 곡	Jeon-Gog
II.3	后溪	Hòuxī	Houhsi	Gokei	후 계	Hu-Gye
II.4	腕骨	Wàngŭ	Wanku	Wankotsu	(수)완골	Su-Wan-Gol
II.5	阳谷	Yánggŭ	Yangku	Yōkoku	양 곡	Yang-Gog
II.6	养老	Yănglăo	Yanglao	Yōrō	양 로	Yang-Ro
II.7	支正	Zhīzhèng	Chihcheng	Shisei	지 정	Ji-Jeong
II.8	小海	Xiăohăi	Hsiaohai	Shōkai	소 해	Yang-So-Hae
II.9	肩贞	Jiānzhēn	Chienchen	Kentei	견 정	Gyeon-Jeong
II.10	臑俞	Nàoshū	Naoshu	Juyu	노 수	No-Su
II.11	天宗	Tiānzōng	Tientsung	Tensō	천 종	Cheon-Jong
II.12	秉风	Bĭngfēng	Pingfeng	Heifū	병 풍	Byeong-Pung
II.13	曲垣	Qūyuán	Chuyuan	Kyokuen	곡 원	Gog-Weon
II.14	肩外俞	Jiānwàishū	Chienwaishu	Kengaiyu	견외수	Gyeon-Oe-Su
II.15	肩中俞	Jiānzhōngshū	Chienchungshu	Kenchūyu	견중수	Gyeon-Jung-Su
II.16	天窗	Tiānchuāng	Tienchuang	Tensō	천 창	Cheon-Chang
II.17	天容	Tiānróng	Tienjung	Tenyō	천 용	Cheon-Yong
II.18	颧髎	Quánliáo	Chuanliao	Kenryō	관 료	Gwan-Ryo
II.19	听宫	Tīnggōng	Tingkung	Chōkyū	청 궁	Cheong-Gung

N = Numbered system · Cc = Han Chinese characters · P = Pinyin Chinese
W = Wade-Giles Chinese · J = Japanese · Kc = Korean characters · K = Korean

F	G	R	V	L
Chao-Tsre	Geringer Teich	Шао-цзэ	Thiêu-trach	Lacus minor
Tsienn-Kou	Vorderes Tal	Цянь-гу	Tién-coc	Vallis anterior
Reou-Tsri	Hintere Schlucht	Хоу-си	Hāu khē	Rivulus posterior
Oann-Kou	Handgelenk-Knochen	Вань-гу	Uyēn-cōt	Foramen carpicum
Iang-Kou	Sonnental	Ян-гу	Duang coc	Vallis yang
Iang-Lao	Pflege des Alters	Ян-лао	Duōng láo	Senectus felix
Tche-Tcheng	Das richtige Glied	Чжи-чжэн	Chi-chánh	Adminiculans orthopathiam
Siao-Rae	Kleines Meer	Сяо-хай	Tieu-hâi	Mare parvum
Tsienn-Tchenn	Schulter-Reinheit	Цзянь-чшэнь	Kien-triuh	Rectum alae
Nao-Iu	Schulter-Punkt	Нао-шу	Nhu du	Inductorium lacerti
Tienn-Tsong	Himmlische Ahnen	Тянь-цзун	Thien tong	Genus caeleste
Tchreng-Fong	Windfahrt	Бин-фэн	Binh phong	Continens ventum
Tsiou-Iuann	Gebogene Mauer	Цюй-юань	Khuc vièn	Murus curvus
Tsienn-Oae	Neben der Schulter	Цзянь-вай-шу	Kiēn ngoai du	Inductorium externum alae
Tsienn-Tchong	Schultermitte	Цзянь-чжун-шу	Kien trung du	Inductorium medium alae
Tsienn-Tchroang	Himmelsfenster	Тянь-чуан	Thiên song	Fenestra caeli
Tienn-Jong	Himmelsfigur	Тянь-жун	Thién dung	Vultus caelestis
Tsiuann-Tsiao	Backenknochengrube	Цюань-ляо	Quyén giao	Cella zygomatica
Ting-Kong	Gehörpalast	Тин-гун	Thinh cung	Conclave auditus

F = French · G = German · R = Russian
V = Vietnamese · L = Latin

Bladder Meridian

N	Cc	P	W	J	Kc	K
III.1	睛明	Jingming	Chingming	Seimei	정 명	Jeong-Myeong
III.2	攒竹	Zǎnzhú	Tsanchu	Sanchiku	찬 죽	Chan-Jug
III.3	眉冲	Méichōng	Meichung	Bishō	미 충	Mi-Chung
III.4	曲差	Qūchāi	Chucha	Kyokusa	곡 차	Gog-Cha
III.5	五处	Wǔchù	Wuchu	Gosho	오 처	O-Cheo
III.6	承光	Chéngguāng	Chengkuang	Shōkō	승 광	Seung-Gwang
III.7	通天	Tōngtiān	Tungtien	Tsūten	통 천	Tong-Cheon
III.8	络却	Luòquè	Lochueh	Rakkyaku	낙 극	Nag-Geug
III.9	玉枕	Yùzhěn	Yuchen	Gyokuchin	옥 침	Og-Chim
III.10	天柱	Tiānzhù	Tienchu	Tenchū	천 주	Cheon-Ju
III.11	大杼	Dàshù	Tachu	Daijo	대 저	Dae-Jeo
III.12	风门	Fēngmén	Fengmen	Fūmon	풍 문	Pung-Mun
III.13	肺俞	Fèishū	Feishu	Haiyu	폐 수	Pye-Su
III.14	厥阴俞	Juéyīnshū	Chuehyinshu	Ketsuinyu	궐음수	Gweol-Eum-Su
III.15	心俞	Xinshū	Hsinshu	Shinyu	심 수	Sim-su
III.16	督俞	Dūshū	Tushu	Tokuyu	독 수	Dog-Su
III.17	膈俞	Géshū	Keshu	Kakuyu	격 수	Gyeog-Su
III.18	肝俞	Gānshū	Kanshu	Kanyu	간 수	Gan-Su
III.19	胆俞	Dǎnshū	Tanshu	Tanyu	담 수	Dam-Su
III.20	脾俞	Pishū	Pishu	Hiyu	비 수	Bi-Su
III.21	胃俞	Wèishū	Weishu	Iyu	위 수	Wi-Su
III.22	三焦俞	Sānjiāoshū	Sanchiaoshu	Sanshōyu	삼초수	Sam-Cho-Su
III.23	肾俞	Shènshū	Shenshu	Jinyu	신 수	Sin-Su

N = Numbered system · Cc = Han Chinese characters · P = Pinyin Chinese
W = Wade-Giles Chinese · J = Japanese · Kc = Korean characters · K = Korean

F	G	R	V	L
Tsing-Ming	Augapfel-Glanz	Цин-мин	Tinh-minh	Canthus nasalis
Tsroann-Tchou	Bambus-Sammeln	Цуань-чжу	Toản-trúc	Stirps supercilii
Mei-Tchrong	Augenbrauen-Passage	Мэй-чун	Mi-xung	Impedimentale supercilii
Tsiou-Tchrae	Gebogene Abweichung	Цюй-ча	Khúc-sai	Impedimentale nasi
Ou-Tchrou	Fünfter Ort	У-чу	Ngủ-xủ	Quinto loco
Tchreng-Koang	Glanz-Vermehrung	Чэн-гуан	Thua-quan	Recipiens luminis
Trong-Tienn	Himmels-Passage	Тун-тянь	Thông-thién	Caelo communicans
Lo-Tsri	LO-Grenze	Лю-цюе	Lac-Khuoc	Nectens recedentem
Iu-Tchenn	Jade-Kissen	Юй-чжень	Ngoc-cham	Cervical iaspidis
Tienn-Tchou	Himmels-Säule	Тянь-чжу	Thiēn-tru	Columna caeli
Ta-Tchrou	Grosses Weberschiffchen	Да-чжу	Dai-trū	Radius magnus
Fong-Menn	Wind-Tor	Фэн-мэнь	Phong-mōn	Porta ventorum
Fei-Iu	Zustimmungspunkt der Lunge	Фэй-шу	Phē-du	Inductorium pulmonale
Tsiue-Inn-Iu	Leere Yin-Punkt	Цзюэ-инь-шу	Khuyét-am-du	Inductorium yin flectentis
Sinn-Iu	Zustimmungspunkt des Herzens	Синь-шу	Tám-du	Inductorium cardiale
Tou-Iu	Zustimmungspunkt des TOU-MO	Ду-шу	Dōc-du	Inductorium regentis
Ko-Iu	Zwerchfellpunkt	Гэ-шу	Cách-du	Inductorium praecordiale
Kann-Iu	Zustimmungspunkt der Leber	Гань-шу	Can-du	Inductorium hepaticum
Tann-Iu	Zustimmungspunkt der Gallenblase	Дань-шу	Dom-du	Inductorium felleum
Pi-Iu	Zustimmungspunkt Milz-Pankreas	Пи-шу	Tỷ-du	Inductorium lienale
Oe-Iu	Zustimmungspunkt des Magens	Вэй-шу	Vi-du	Inductorium stomachi
Sann-Tsiao-Iu	Zustimmungspunkt des "Dreifachen Erwärmers"	Сань-цзяо-шу	Tam-tieu-du	Inductorium tricalorii
Chenn-Iu	Zustimmungspunkt der Niere	Шэнь-шу	Than-du	Inductorium renale

F = French · G = German · R = Russian
V = Vietnamese · L = Latin

N	Cc	P	W	J	Kc	K
III.24	气海俞	Qihǎishū	Chihaishu	Kikaiyu	기해수	Gi-Hae-Su
III.25	大肠俞	Dàchángshū	Tachangshu	Daichōyu	대장수	Dae-Jang-Su
III.26	关元俞	Guānyuánshū	Kuanyuanshu	Kangenyu	관원수	Gwan-Weon-Su
III.27	小肠俞	Xiǎochángshū	Hsiaochangshu	Shōchōyu	소장수	So-Jang-Su
III.28	膀胱俞	Pangguāngshū	Pangkuangshu	Bōkōyu	방광수	Bang-Gwang-Su
III.29	中膂俞	Zhōnglǔshū	Chunglushu	Chūryoyu	중려수	Jung-Lyeo-Su
III.30	白环俞	Baihuánshū	Paihuanshu	Hakkanyu	백환수	Baeg-Hwan-Su
III.31	上髎	Shàngliáo	Shangliao	Jōryō	상 료	Sang-Ryo
III.32	次髎	Cìliáo	Tzuliao	Jiryō	차 료	Cha-Ryo
III.33	中髎	Zhōngliáo	Chungliao	Chūryō	중 료	Jung-Ryo
III.34	下髎	Xiàliáo	Hsialiao	Geryō	하 료	Ha-Ryo
III.35	会阳	Huìyáng	Huiyang	Eyō	회 양	Hoe-Yang
III.36/41	附分	Fùfēn	Fufen	Fubun	부 분	Bu-Bun
III.37/42	魄户	Pòhù	Pohu	Hakko	백 호	Baeg-Ho
III.38/43	膏肓	Gāohuāng	Kaohuang	Kōkō	고 황	Go-Hwang
III.39/44	神堂	Shéntáng	Shentang	Shindō	신 당	Sin-Dang
III.40/45	譩譆	Yixi	Yihsi	Iki	의 희	Eui-Heui
III.41/46	膈关	Géguān	Kekuan	Kakkan	격 관	Gyeog-Gwan
III.42/47	魂门	Húnmén	Hunmen	Konmon	혼 문	Hon-Mun
III.43/48	阳纲	Yánggāng	Yangkang	Yōkō	양 강	Yang-Gang
III.44/49	意舍	Yishè	Yishe	Isha	의 사	Eui-Sa
III.45/50	胃仓	Wèicāng	Weitsang	Isō	위 창	Wi-Chang
III.46/51	肓门	Huāngmén	Huangmen	Kōmon	황 문	Hwang-Mun

N = Numbered system · Cc = Han Chinese characters · P = Pinyin Chinese
W = Wade-Giles Chinese · J = Japanese · Kc = Korean characters · K = Korean

F	G	R	V	L
Tsri-Rae-Iu	Punkt des Atem-Meeres	Ци-хай-шу	Khi-hai-du	Inductorium maris ch'i
Ta-Tchrang-Iu	Zustimmungspunkt des Dickdarms	Да-чан-шу	Dai-truong-du	Inductorium intestini crassi
Koann-Iuann-Iu	Punkt des Grenz-Ursprungs	Гуань-юань-шу	Quan-nguyēn-du	Inductorium prima clusarum
Siao-Tchrang-Iu	Zustimmungspunkt des Dunndarms	Сяо-чан-шу	Tieu-truong-du	Inductorium intestini tenuis
Prang-Koang-Iu	Zustimmungspunkt der Harnblase	Пан-гуань-шу	Ban-quang-du	Inductorium vesicale
Tchong-Liu-Iu	Zustimmungspunkt der mittleren Wirbelkörper	Чжун-люй-шу	Trung-lú-du	Inductorium pro medio tergo
Pae-Roann-Iu	Punkt des Sphinkters	Бай-хуань-шу	Bach-hoan-du	Inductorium anuli candidi
Chang-Tsiao	Obere Grube	Шан-ляо	Thuong-liēu	Cella superior
Tsre-Tsiao	Folgende Grube	Цы-ляо	Thu-liēn	Cella secunda
Tchong-Tsiao	Mittlere Grube	Чжун-ляо	Trung-lieu	Cella media
Sia-Tsiao	Untere Grube	Ся-ляо	Ha-lieu	Cella inferior
Roe-Iang	Yang-Vereinung	Хуэй-ян	Hôi-duong	Yang conventi
Fou-Fenn	Neben dem Muskel	Чэн-фу	Phu-phan	Pars addita
Pro-Rou	Sitz der Seele	Инь-мэнь	Phach-ho	Ostium animae
Kao-Roang	Lebenszentren	Фу-си	Cao-hoang	Venae et viscera
Chenn-Trang	Göttliche Halle	Вэй-ян	Than-duong	Atrium shen
I-Si	Schmerzensschrei	Вэй-чжун	Y-hi	Exoptatum!
Ko-Koann	Zwerchfellgrenze	Фу-фэнь	Cach-quan	Clusa praecordialis
Roun-Menn	Tor der Geisterseele	По-ху	Hòn-mon	Porta animi
Iang-Kang	Yang-Bindung	Гао-хуан	Duong-cuong	Generale yang
I-Che	Gefühls-Sitz	Шэн-тан	Y-xả	Domus phantasiae
Oe-Tsrang	Magenspeicher	И-си	Vi-thuong	Granarium stomachi
Roang-Menn	Tor der Lebenszentren	Гэ-гуань	Manh-môn	Porta viscerum

F = French · G = German · R = Russian
V = Vietnamese · L = Latin

N	Cc	P	W	J	Kc	K
III.47/52	志室	Zhìshì	Chihshih	Shishitsu	지 실	Ji-Sil
III.48/53	胞肓	Bāohuāng	Paohuang	Hōkō	포 황	Po-Hwang
III.49/54	秩边	Zhìbiān	Chihpien	Chippen	질 변	Jil-Byeon
III.50/36	承扶	Chéngfú	Chengfu	Shōfu	승 부	Seung-Bu
III.51/37	殷门	Yīnmén	Yinmen	Inmon	은 문	Eun-Mun
III.52/38	浮郄	Fúxi	Fuhsi	Fugeki	부 극	Bu-Geug
III.53/39	委阳	Wěiyáng	Weiyang	Iyō	위 양	Wi-Yang
III.54/40	委中	Wěizhōng	Weichung	Ichū	위 중	Wi-Jung
III.55	合阳	Héyáng	Heyang	Gōyō	합 양	Hab-Yang
III.56	承筋	Chéngjīn	Chengchin	Shōkin	승 근	Seung-Geun
III.57	承山	Chéngshān	Chengshan	Shōzan	승 산	Seung-San
III.58	飞扬	Fēiyáng	Feiyang	Hiyō	비 양	Bi-Yang
III.59	跗阳	Fūyáng	Fuyang	Fuyō	부 양	Bu-Yang
III.60	昆仑	Kūnlún	Kunlun	Konron	곤 륜	Gon-Ryun
III.61	仆参	Púshēn	Pushen	Bokushin	복 삼	Bog-Sam
III.62	申脉	Shēnmài	Shenmo	Shinmyaku	신 맥	Sin-Maeg
III.63	金门	Jīnmén	Chinmen	Kinmon	금 문	Geum-Mun
III.64	京骨	Jīnggǔ	Chingku	Keikotsu	경 골	Gyeong-Gol
III.65	束骨	Shùgǔ	Shuku	Sokkotsu	속 골	Sog-Gol
III.66	通谷	Tonggu	Tsu tungku	Ashi no Tsūkoku	(족)통곡	Jog-Tong-Gog
III.67	至阴	Zhiyīn	Chihyin	Shiin	지 음	Ji-Eum

N = Numbered system · Cc = Han Chinese characters · P = Pinyin Chinese
W = Wade-Giles Chinese · J = Japanese · Kc = Korean characters · K = Korean

F	G	R	V	L
Tche-Che	Willens-Sitz	Хунь-мэнь	Chi-that	Conclave potentiae
Pao-Roang	Lebenszentren der Gebärmutter	Ян-ган	Bao-manh	Viscera involuta
Tche-Pienn	Seite des 4. Wirbels	И-шэ	Trat-bièn	Margo subsequens
Tchreng-Fou	Halt der Stütze	Вэй-цан	Thua-pho	Rima carnis
Inn-Menn	Reichtums-Tor	Хуан-мэнь	An-mon	Porta femoris
Feou-Tsri	Oberflächliches Tal	Чжи-ши	Phu-ky	Rima superficialis
Oe-Iang	Yang-Speicherung	Бао-хуан	Uy-duong	Yang lacunae
Oe-Tchong	Mittlere Speicherung	Чжи-бянь	Uy-trung	Medium lacunae
Ro-Iang	Treffpunkt des Yang	Хэ-ян	Hiep-duong	Yang coniuncti
Tchreng-Tsinn	Musket-Stütze	Чэн-цзинь	Thùa-căn	Recipiens nervos
Tchreng-Chann	Berg-Stütze	Чэн-шань	Thua son	Columna carnis
Fei-Iang	Aufschwung	Фэй-ян	Phi-duong	Yang flectens
Fou-Iang	Yang des Fussknochens	Фу-ян	Phu-duong	Yang tarsi
Kroun-Loun	Name eines Berges in Tibet	Кунь-лунь	Con-lon	Olympus
Prou-Chenn	Hilfe des Hausangestallten	Пу-шэнь	Bot-tham	Servi salutatio
Chenn-Mo	Gefäss-Streckung	Шэнь-май	Thān-mach	Origo ascendentis yang
Tsinn-Menn	Gold-Tor	Цзинь-мэнь	Kim-mōn	Porta metalli
Tsing-Kou	Haupt-Knochen	Цзин-гу	Kinh-ćot	Os pyramidale
Chou-Kou	Knochen-Bindung	Шу-гу	Thut-cōt	Os ligatum
Trong-Kou	Tal-Passage	Тун-гу	Thōng-coc	Vallis communicans vesicalis
Tche-Inn	Erreichung des Yin	Чжи-инь	Chi-ām	Yin supremum

F = French · G = German · R = Russian
V = Vietnamese · L = Latin

Kidney Meridian

N	Cc	P	W	J	Kc	K
IV.1	涌泉	Yǒngquán	Yungchuan	Yūsen	용 천	Yong-Cheon
IV.2	然谷	Rángǔ	Janku	Nenkoku	연 곡	Yeon-Gog
IV.3	太溪	Tàixī	Taihsi	Taikei	태 계	Tae-Gye
IV.4	大钟	Dàzhōng	Tachung	Daishō	대 종	Dae-Jong
IV.5	水泉	Shuǐquán	Shuichuan	Suisen	수 천	Su-Cheon
IV.6	照海	Zhàohǎi	Chaohai	Shōkai	조 해	Jo-Hae
IV.7	复溜	Fùliū	Fuliu	Fukuryū	부 류	Bu-Ryu
IV.8	交信	Jiāoxìn	Chiaohsin	Kōshin	교 신	Gyo-sin
IV.9	筑宾	Zhùbīn	Chupin	Chikuhin	축 빈	Chug-Bin
IV.10	阴谷	Yīngǔ	Yinku	Inkoku	음 곡	Eum-Gog
IV.11	横骨	Hénggǔ	Hengku	Ōkotsu	횡 골	Hoeng-Gol
IV.12	大赫	Dàhè	Taheh	Daikaku	대 혁	Dae-Hyeog
IV.13	气穴	Qixué	Chihsueh	Kiketsu	기 혈	Gi-Hyeol
IV.14	四满	Simǎn	Szuman	Shiman	사 만	Sa-Man
IV.15	中注	[Abdomen] Zhōngzhù	Chungchu	Chūchū	중 주	Jung-Ju
IV.16	肓俞	Huāngshū	Huangshu	Kōyu	황 수	Hwang-Su
IV.17	商曲	Shāngqū	Shangchu	Shōkyoku	상 곡	Sang-Gog
IV.18	石关	Shíguān	Shihkuan	Sekikan	석 관	Seog-Gwan
IV.19	阴都	Yindū	Yintu	Into	음 도	Eum-Do
IV.20	通谷	[Abdomen] Tonggu	Fu Tungku	Hara no Tsūkoku	(복)통곡	Bog-Tong-Gog
IV.21	幽门	Yōumén	Yumen	Yūmon	유 문	Yu-Mun
IV.22	步廊	Bùláng	Pulang	Horō	보 랑	Bo-Rang
IV.23	神封	Shēnfēng	Shenfeng	Shimpō	신 봉	Sin-Bong
IV.24	灵墟	Lingxū	Linghsu	Reikyo	영 허	Yeong-Heo
IV.25	神藏	Shéncáng	Shentsang	Shinzō	신 장	Sin-Jang
IV.26	彧中	Yùzhōng	Yuchung	Wakuchū	욱 중	Ug-Jung
IV.27	俞府	Shūfǔ	Shufu	Yufu	수 부	Su-Bu

N = Numbered system · Cc = Han Chinese characters · P = Pinyin Chinese
W = Wade-Giles Chinese · J = Japanese · Kc = Korean characters · K = Korean

F	G	R	V	L
Iong-Tsiuann	Sprudelnde Quelle	Юн-цюань	Dũng-tuyẽn	Fons scatens
Jenn-Kou	Das Tal der Bewährung	Жань-гу	Nhien-cöc	Fons draconis
Trae-Tsri	Leucht-Meer	Тай-си	Thái-khé	Rivulus maior
Ta-Tchong	Wasser-Quelle	Да-чжун	Dai-chung	Campana magna
Choe-Tsiuann	Höchste Schlucht	Шуй-цюань	Thùy-tuyën	Fons aquarum
Tchao-Rae	Gross-Becher	Чжао-хай	Phuc luu	Mare illustratum
Fou-Leou	Hinterer Strom	Фу-лю	Chiëu-hài	Amnis recurrens
Tsiao-Sinn	Wechselvielseitiges Vertrauen	Цзяо-синь	Giao-tin	Cursores copulati
Tso-Pinn	Deich-Bau	Чжу-бин	Chuc-tan	Ripa spissa
Inn-Kou	Yin-Tal	Инь-гу	Âm-cöc	Vallis yin
Rong-Kou	Quer-Knochen	Хэн-гу	Hoǎnh-cöt	Os transversum
Ta-Ro	Gross-Glanz	Да-хэ	Dai-hich	Clusa yin
Tsri-Tsiue	Punkt der Energie	Ци-сюе	Khi-huyêt	Foramen ch'i
Se-Mann	Vierfache Fülle	Сы-мань	Tú-mān	Plenum quartum
Tchong-Tchou	Mittlerer Fluss	Чжун-чжу	Trung-chú	Infusio media
Roang-Iu	Zustimmungspunkt der Lebenszentren	Хуан-шу	Manh-du	Inductorium viscerum
Chang-Tsiou	Wendeplatz der Kaufleute	Шан-цюй	Thuong-khuc	Curvatura alta
Che-Koann	Stein-Grenze	Ши-гуань	Thach-quang	Clusa lapidea
Inn-Tou	Hauptstadt des Yin	Инь-ду	Âm-dô	Urbs yin
Trong-Kou	Tal-Passage	Фу-тун-гу	Thong-coc	Vallis communicans renalis
Iou-Menn	Dunkel-Tor	Ю-мэнь	U-mon	Porta pylorica
Pou-Lang	Veranda-Beschreitung	Бу-лан	Bô-lang	Porticus peripatetica
Chenn-Fong	Götter-Siegel	Шэнь-фэн	Thän-phong	Altare shen
Ling-Siu	Geist-Leere	Лин-сюй	Linh-khuu	Vacuitas responsiva
Chenn-Tsrang	Götter-Speicher	Шэнь-цан	Thän-tang	Horreum shen
Rouo-Tchong	In dem Zweifel	Юй-чжун	Hoac-trung	In terra nostra
Iu-Fou	Werkstatt der Zustimmung	Шу-фу	Du-phù	Aula inductoria

F = French · G = German · R = Russian
V = Vietnamese · L = Latin

Circulation–sex

N	Cc	P	W	J	Kc	K
V.1	天池	Tiānchí	Tienchih	Tenchi	천 지	Cheon-Ji
V.2	天泉	Tiānquán	Tienchuan	Tensen	천 천	Cheon-Cheon
V.3	曲泽	Qūzé	Chutse	Kyokutaku	곡 택	Gog-Taeg
V.4	郄门	Xìmén	Hsimen	Gekimon	극 문	Geug-Mun
V.5	间使	Jiānshǐ	Chienshih	Kanshi	간 사	Gan-Sa
V.6	内关	Nèiguān	Neikuan	Naikan	내 관	Nae-Kwan
V.7	大陵	Dàlíng	Taling	Dairyō	대 릉	Dae-Leung
V.8	劳宫	Láogōng	Laokung	Rōkyū	노 궁	No-Gung
V.9	中冲	Zhōngchōng	Chungchung	Chūshō	중 충	Jung-Chung

N = Numbered system · Cc = Han Chinese characters · P = Pinyin Chinese
W = Wade-Giles Chinese · J = Japanese · Kc = Korean characters · K = Korean

F	G	R	V	L
Tienn-Tchre	Himmels-Teich	Тянь-чи	Thiēn-tri	Stagnum caeleste
Tienn-Tsiuann	Himmels-Quelle	Тянь-цюань	Thiēn-tuyēn	Fons caelestis
Tsiou-Tsre	Gewundener Teich	Цюй-цзэ	Khúc-trach	Lacus curvus
Tsri-Menn	Grenz-Tor	Си-мэнь	Ky-m̄on	Porta rimica
Tsienn-Che	Der Zwischengesandte	Цзянь-ми	Gian-sū	Foramen intermedium
Nei-Koann	Innen-Grenze	Нэй-гуань	Nōi-quang	Clusa interna
Ta-Ling	Gross-Hügel	Да-лин	Dai-lang	Tumulus magnus
Lao-Kong	Palast der Mühen	Лао-гун	Lao-cung	Medium palmae
Tchong-Tchrong	Mittlerer Angriffspunkt	Чжун-чун	Trung-xung	Impedimentale medium

F = French · G = German · R = Russian
V = Vietnamese · L = Latin

Three Heater Meridian

N	Cc	P	W	J	Kc	K
VI.1	关冲	Guānchōng	Kuanchong	Kansyō	관 충	Gwan-Chung
VI.2	液门	Yèmén	Yemen	Ekimon	액 문	Aeg-Mun
VI.3	中渚	Zhōngzhǔ	Chungchu	Chūsho	중 저	Jung-Jeo
VI.4	阳池	Yángchí	Yangchih	Yōchi	양 지	Yang-Ji
VI.5	外关	Wàiguān	Waikuan	Gaikan	외 관	Oe-Gwan
VI.6	支沟	Zhīgōu	Chihkou	Shikō	지 구	Ji-Gu
VI.7	会宗	Huizōng	Huitsung	Esō	회 종	Hoe-Jong
VI.8	三阳络	Sānyángluò	Sanyanglo	Sanyōraku	삼양락	Sam-Yang-Rag
VI.9	四渎	Sìdú	Szutu	Shitoku	사 독	Sa-Dog
VI.10	天井	Tiānjǐng	Tienching	Tensei	천 정	Cheon-Jeong
VI.11	清冷渊	Qīnglěngyuān	Chinglengyuan	Seireien	청랭연	Cheong-Raeng-Yeon
VI.12	消泺	Xiāoluò	Hsiaolo	Shōreki	소 락	So-Rag
VI.13	臑会	Nàohuì	Naohui	Jue	노 회	No-Hoe
VI.14	肩髎	Jiānliáo	Chienliao	Kenryō	견 료	Gyeon-Ryo
VI.15	天髎	Tiānliáo	Tienliao	Tenryō	천 료	Cheon-Ryo
VI.16	天牖	Tiānyǒu	Tienyu	Tenyū	천 유	Cheon-Yu
VI.17	翳风	Yifēng	Yifeng	Eifū	예 풍	Ye-Pung
VI.18	瘈脉	Qìmài	Chihmo	Keimyaku	계 맥	Gye-Maeg
VI.19	颅息	Lúxī	Luhsi	Rosoku	노 식	No-Sig
VI.20	角孙	Jiǎosūn	Chuehsun	Kakuson	각 손	Gag-Son
VI.21	耳门	Ěrmén	Erhmen	Jimon	이 문	I-Mun
VI.22	和髎	[Ear] Heliao	Holiao	Waryō	(이)화료	I-Hwa-Ryo
VI.23	丝竹空	Sizhúkōng	Ssuchukung	Shichikukū	사죽공	Sa-Jug-Gong

N = Numbered system · Cc = Han Chinese characters · P = Pinyin Chinese
W = Wade-Giles Chinese · J = Japanese · Kc = Korean characters · K = Korean

F	G	R	V	L
Koann-Tchrong	Grenz-Angriffs-Punkt	Гуань-чун	Quan-xung	Impedimentale clusae
Ie-Menn	Flüssigkeits-Tor	Е-мэнь	Dich-mōn	Porta suci
Tchong-Tchou	Mittel-Insel	Чжун-чжу	Trung-chu	Insula media
Iang-Tchre	Yang-Teich	Ян-чи	Duong-tri	Stagnum yang
Oae-Koann	Aussen-Grenze	Вай-гуань	Ngoai-quan	Clusa externa
Tche-Keou	Zweiggraben	Чжи-гоу	Chi-cáu	Tigris volans
Roe-Tsong	Begegnung mit den Ahnen	Хуэй-цзун	Hôi-tông	Genus conventum
Sann-Iang-Lo	LO der 3 Yang	Сань-ян-ло	Tam-duong-lac	Porta communicans
Se-Tou	4 Wasserläufe	Сы-ду	Tú-dôc	Quattuor incilium
Tienn-Tsing	Himmels-Brunnen	Тянь-цзинь	Thiēn-tinh	Puteus caelestis
Tsring-Ling-Iuann	Klarkühler-Wasserstrudel	Цин-лэн-юань	Thanh-lānh-uyên	Fons limpidus ac frigidus
Siao-Lo	Ableitung des stagnierenden Wassers	Сяо-лэ	Tiêu-lac	Quod dispellit
Nao-Roe	Oberarm-Punkt	Нао-хуэй	Nhu-hôi	Conventus lacerti
Tsienn-Tsiao	Schulter-Grube	Цзянь-ляо	Kiên-liêu	Cella alae
Tsienn-Tsiao	Himmels-Grube	Тянь-ляо	Thien-lieu	Cella caelestis
Tienn-Iou	Himmels-Gitterfenster	Тянь-ю	Thiên-dú	Apertura caeli
I-Fong	Windschirm	И-фэн	Ë-phong	Pluteus venti
Tchre-Mo	Pulsierende Ader	Ци-май	Khë-mach	Foramen spasticum
Lou-Si	Schädelatmung	Лу-си	Lu-tuc	Auriculare posterius
Tsio-Soun	Absteigen von der Ohrspitze	Цзяо-сунь	Giác-tôn	Temporale superius
Se-Tchou-Kong	Seidenbambus	Эр-мэнь	Tu-truc-không	Porta auris
Ro-Tsiao	Korngrube der Schläfen	Хэ-ляо	Hoà-lieu	Cella harmoniae
El-Menn	Ohr-Tor	Сы-чжу-кун	Nhi-mōn	Fides et fistulae

F = French · G = German · R = Russian
V = Vietnamese · L = Latin

Gall Bladder Meridian

N	Cc	P	W	J	Kc	K
VII.1	瞳子髎	Tóngzǐliáo	Tungtzuliao	Dōshiryō	동자료	Dong-Ja-Ryo
VII.2	听会	Tīnghuì	Tinghui	Chōe	청 회	Chong-Hoe
VII.3	上关	Shàngguān	Shangkuan	Kakushujin	(상관)	Gaeg-Ju-In
VII.4	颔厌	Hànyàn	Hanyen	Ganen	함 염	Ham-Yeom
VII.5	悬颅	Xuánlú	Hsuanlu	Kenro	현 로	Hyeon-Ro
VII.6	悬厘	Xuánli	Hsuanli	Kenri	현 리	Hyeon-Ri
VII.7	曲鬓	Qūbìn	Chupin	Kyokubin	곡 빈	Gog-Bin
VII.8	率谷	Shuàigǔ	Shuaiku	Sokkoku	솔 곡	Sol-Gog
VII.9	天冲	Tiānchōng	Tienchung	Tenshō	천 충	Cheon-Chung
VII.10	浮白	Fúbái	Fupai	Fuhaku	부 백	Bu-Baeg
VII.11	窍阴	[Head] Qiaoyin	Tou chiaoyin	Atama no Kyōin	(두)규음	Du-Gyu-Eum
VII.12	完骨	[Head] Wángǔ	Wanku	Kankotsu	(두)완골	Du-Wan-Gol
VII.13	本神	Běnshén	Penshen	Honshin	본 신	Bon-Sin
VII.14	阳白	Yángbái	Yangpai	Yōhaku	양 백	Yang-Baeg
VII.15	头临泣	[Head] Linqi	Tou Linchi	Atama no Rinkyū	(두)임읍	Du-Im-Eub
VII.16	目窗	Mùchuāng	Muchuang	Mokusō	목 창	Mog-Chang
VII.17	正营	Zhèngyíng	Chengying	Shōei	정 영	Jeong-Yeong
VII.18	承灵	Chénglíng	Chengling	Shōrei	승 령	Seung-Lyeong
VII.19	脑空	Nǎokōng	Naokung	Nōkū	뇌 공	Noe-Gong
VII.20	风池	Fēngchí	Fengchih	Fūchi	풍 지	Pung-Ji
VII.21	肩井	Jiānjǐng	Chienching	Kensei	견 정	Dam-Gyeon-Jeong
VII.22	渊腋	Yuānyè	Yuanyeh	Eneki	연 액	Yeon-Aeg
VII.23	辄筋	Zhéjīn	Chechin	Chōkin	첩 근	Cheob-Geun

N = Numbered system · Cc = Han Chinese characters · P = Pinyin Chinese
W = Wade-Giles Chinese · J = Japanese · Kc = Korean characters · K = Korean

F	G	R	V	L
Trong-Tse-Tsiao	Pupillen-Grube	Тун-цзы-ляо	Dōng-tù-liêu	Cella pupillae
Ting-Roe	Gehörs-Punkt	Тин-хуэй	Thinh-hôi	Conventus auditus
Kro-Tchou-Jenn	Gast und Hausherr	Шан-гуань	Khách-chū-nhon	Clusa superior
Rann-Ia	Kinnbacken-Drücker	Хань-янь	Hàm-yëm	In angulo sphenoidalis
Siuann-Lou	Stirnüberhang	Сюань-лу	Huyen-lu	Foramen medullae
Siuann-Li	Die Freischwebende Balance	Сюань-ли	Huyēn-ly	Lobulus suspensus
Tsiou-Ping	Gewundenes Schläfenhaar	Цюй-бинь	Khúc-män	Curvatura coruli
Choae-Kou	Das Ende des Tales	Шуай-гу	Suat-coc	Apex auriculi
Tienn-Tchrong	Himmels-Punkt	Тянь-чун	Bòn-thän	Impedimentale caeleste
Feou-Pae	Flutende Helle	Фу-бай	Duong-bach	Candor superficialis
Tsiao-Inn	Yin des Anfangs	Тоу-цяо-инь	Lâm-khāp	Yin penetrans capitis
Oann-Kou	Vollendeter Knochen	Вань-гу	Muc-song	Processus mastoideus
Penn-Chenn	Ursprungs-Geist	Бэнь-шень	Khiĕu-am	Shen stirpis
Iang-Pae	Entfaltung des Hellen	Ян-бай	Thua-linh	Candor yang
Linn-Tsri	Tränen-Abstieg	Тоу-линь-ци	Thiên-xung	Lacrimarum instantium capitis
Mou-Tchroang	Augenfenster	Му-чуан	Phu-bach	Fenestra oculi
Tcheng-Ing	Rechte Leitung	Чжэн-ин	Hoan-cöt	Castra praetoriana
Tchreng-Ling	Geist-Empfang	Чэн-лин	Chánh-dinh	Recipiens vis responsiva
Nao-Krong	Gehirn-Raum	Нао-кун	Nāo-không	Hiatus cerebri
Fong-Tchre	Wind-Teich	Фэн-чи	Phong-tri	Stagnum venti
Tienn-Tsing	Schulter-Brunnen	Цзянь-цзин	Kiên-tinh	Puteus alae
Iuann-Ie	Strudel-Wasser	Юань-е	Uyên-dich	Porta axillae
Tchre-Tsinn	Flanken-Muskel	Чжэ-цзинь	Tiëp-can	Atrium axillae

F = French · G = German · R = Russian
V = Vietnamese · L = Latin

N	Cc	P	W	J	Kc	K
VII.24	日月	Riyuè	Jihyueh	Jitsugetsu	일 월	Il-Weol
VII.25	京门	Jīngmén	Chingmen	Keimon	경 문	Gyeong-Mun
VII.26	带脉	Dàimài	Taimo	Taimyaku	대 맥	Dae-Maeg
VII.27	五枢	Wŭshū	Wushu	Gosū	오 추	O-Chu
VII.28	维道	Wéidào	Weitao	Idō	유 도	Yu-Do
VII.29	居髎	[Femur] Jūliáo	Chuliao	Kyoryō	(고)거료	Go-Geo-Ryo
VII.30	环跳	Huántiào	Huantiao	Kanchō	환 조	Hwan-Jo
VII.31	风市	Fēngshì	Fengshih	Fūshi	풍 시	Pung-Si
VII.32	中渎	[Femur] Zhōngdú	Chungtu	Chūtoku	중 독	Jung-Dog
VII.33	膝阳关	Xīyángguān	Tsu Yangkuan	Ashi no Yōkan	양 관	Seul-Yang-Gwan
VII.34	阳陵泉	Yánglingquán	Yanglingchuan	Yōryōsen	양릉천	Yang-Leung-Cheon
VII.35	阳交	Yángjiāo	Yangchiao	Yōkō	양 교	Yang-Gyo
VII.36	外丘	Wàiqiū	Waichiu	Gaikyū	외 구	Oe-Gu
VII.37	光明	Guāngmíng	Kuangming	Kōmei	광 명	Gwang-Myeong
VII.38	阳辅	Yángfŭ	Yangfu	Yōho	양 보	Yang-Bo
VII.39	悬钟	Xuánzhōng	Hsuanchung	Kenshō	현 종	Hyeon-Jong
VII.40	丘墟	Qiūxū	Chiuhsu	Kyūkyo	구 허	Gu-Heo
VII.41	足临泣	[Foot] Linqì	Tsu Linchi	Ashi no Rinkyū	(족)임읍	Jog-Im-Eub
VII.42	地五会	Dìwŭhuì	Tiwuhui	Chigoe	지오회	Ji-O-Hoe
VII.43	侠溪	Xiáxī	Hsiahsi	Kyōkei	협 계	Hyeob-Gye
VII.44	足窍阴	[Foot] Qiàoyīn	Tsu Chiaoyin	Ashi no Kyōin	(족)규음	Jog-Gyu-Eum

N = Numbered system · Cc = Han Chinese characters · P = Pinyin Chinese
W = Wade-Giles Chinese · J = Japanese · Kc = Korean characters · K = Korean

F	G	R	V	L
Je-Iue	Sonne-Mond	Жи-юе	Nhut-nguyét	Sol et luna
Tsing-Menn	Haupstadt-Tor	Цзин-мэнь	Kinh-môn	Porta pyramidis
Tae-Mo	Gürtel-Gefäss	Дай-май	Dái-mach	Foramen sinarteriae zonalis
Ou-Tchrou	Fünf Zentralpfeiler	У-шу	Ngū-xu	Cardo quintus
Oe-Tao	Verbindungsweg	Вэй-дао	Duy-dao	Via retinentis
Tsiu-Tsiao	Ruhe-Grube	Цзюй-ляо	Cu-liêu	Cella habitationis
Roann-Tsiao	In den Reifen springen	Хуань-тяо	Hoan-khiêu	Cardo femoralis
Fong-Che	Wind-Markt	Фэн-ши	Phong-thi	Forum ventorum
Sia-Tou	Unterer Wasserlauf	Чжун-ду	Trung-dôc	Incile medium
Iang-Koann	Yang-Grenze	Цзу-ян-гуань	Duong-quang	Clusa yang fellea
Iang-Ling-Tsiuann	Yang-Hügel-Quelle	Ян-лин-цюань	Duong-lăng	Fons tumuli yang
Iang-Tsiao	Yang-Treffpunkt	Ян-цзяо	Duong-giao	Copulatio yang
Cae-Tsiou	Aussen-Hügel	Вай-цю	Ngoai-khuu	Monticulus externus
Koang-Ming	Strahlende Helle	Гуан-мин	Quang-minh	Lumen ac splendor
Iang-Fou	Stütze des Yang	Ян-фу	Duong-phù	Divisio carnis
Siuann-Tchong	Aufgehängte Glocke	Сюань-чжун	Huven-chung	Campana suspensa
Tsiou-Siu	Hügel-Markt	Цю-сюй	Khuu-hu	Agger monticuli
Linn-Tsri	Tränen-Abstieg	Цзу-линь-ци	Túc-lâm-khăp	Lacrimarum instantium pedis
Ti-Ou-Roe	Fünfte Vereinigung der Erde	Ди-у-хуэй	Dia-ngù-hôi	Conventus quintus terrae
Sie-Tsri	Verengtes Tal	Ся-си	Hiêp-khê	Rivulus coercitus
Tsiao-Inn	Yin des Anfangs	Цзу-цяо-инь	Túc-khiêu-âm	Yin penetrans pedis

F = French · G = German · R = Russian
V = Vietnamese · L = Latin

Liver Meridian

N	Cc	P	W	J	Kc	K
VIII.1	大敦	Dàdūn	Tatun	Daiton	대 돈	Dae-Don
VIII.2	行间	Xingjiān	Hsingchien	Kōkan	행 간	Haeng-Gan
VIII.3	太冲	Tàichōng	Taichung	Taishō	태 충	Tae-Chung
VIII.4	中封	Zhōngfēng	Chungfeng	Chūhō	중 봉	Jung-Bong
VIII.5	蠡沟	Ligōu	Likou	Reikō	여 구	Yeo-Gu
VIII.6	中都	Zhōngdū	Chungtu	Chūto	중 도	Jung-Do
VIII.7	膝关	Xīguān	Hsikuan	Shitsukan	슬 관	Seul-Gwan
VIII.8	曲泉	Qūquán	Chuchuan	Kyokusen	곡 천	Gog-Cheon
VIII.9	阴包	Yīnbāo	Yinpao	Impō	음 포	Eum-Po
VIII.10	五里	[Femur] Wuli	Tsuwuli	Ashi no Gori	(각)오리	Gag-O-Ri
VIII.11	阴廉	Yīnlián	Yinlien	Inren	음 렴	Eum-Ryeom
VIII.12	急脉	Jímài	Chimo	Kyūmyaku	급 맥	Geub-Maeg
VIII.13	章门	Zhāngmén	Changmen	Shōmon	장 문	Jang-Mun
VIII.14	期门	Qīmén	Chimen	Kimon	기 문	Bog-Gi-Mun

N = Numbered system · Cc = Han Chinese characters · P = Pinyin Chinese
W = Wade-Giles Chinese · J = Japanese · Kc = Korean characters · K = Korean

F	G	R	V	L
Ta-Toun	Grosse Aufrichtigkeit	Да-дунь	Dai-dôn	Lanx magna
Sing-Tsienn	Gang-Strecke	Син-цзянь	Hanh-gian	Interstitium ambulatorium
Trae-Tchrong	Höchster Angriffspunkt	Тай-чун	Thai-xung	Impedimentale maius
Tchong-Fong	Mitte-Siegel	Чжун-фэн	Trung-phong	Altare medium
Li-Keou	Endrinne	Ли-гоу	Lây-cău	Canalis teredinis
Tchong-Tou	Stadt der Mitte	Чжун-ду	Trung-dò	Urbs media
Si-Koann	Knie-Grenze	Ци-гуань	Tät-quang	Clusa genus
Tsiou-Tsiuann	Gebogene Quelle	Цюй-цюань	Khúc-tuyën	Fons curvus
Inn-Pao	Yin-Hülle	Инь-бао	Am-bào	Foramen uteri
Ou-Li	Fünf-Li	Цзу-у-ли	Ngú-lý	Vicus quintus pedis
Inn-Lienn	Yin-Winkel	Инь-лянь	Âm-lièm	Angustiae yin
Iang-Che	Schaf-Pfeil	Цзи-май	Cäp-mach	Pulsus excitatus
Tchang-Menn	Gesetzes-Tor	Чжан-мэнь	Chuong-môn	Conquisitorium lienale
Tsri-Menn	Zeit-Tor	Ци-мэнь	Kỳ-môn	Conquisitorium hepaticum

F = French · G = German · R = Russian
V = Vietnamese · L = Latin

Lung Meridian

N	Cc	P	W	J	Kc	K
IX.1	中府	Zhōngfǔ	Chungfu	Chūfu	중 부	Jung-Bu
IX.2	云门	Yúnmén	Yunmen	Unmon	운 문	Un-Mun
IX.3	天府	Tiānfǔ	Tienfu	Tempu	천 부	Cheon-Bu
IX.4	侠白	Xiábái	Hsiapai	Kyōhaku	협 백	Hyeob-Baeg
IX.5	尺泽	Chǐzé	Chihtse	Shakutaku	척 택	Cheog-Taeg
IX.6	孔最	Kǒngzuì	Kungtsui	Kōsai	공 최	Gong-Choe
IX.7	列缺	Lièquē	Liehchueh	Rekketsu	열 결	Yeol-Gyeol
IX.8	经渠	Jīngqú	Chingchu	Keikyo	경 거	Gyeong-Geo
IX.9	太渊	Tàiyuān	Taiyuan	Taien	태 연	Tae-Yeon
IX.10	鱼际	Yújì	Yuchi	Gyosai	어 제	Eo-Je
IX.11	少商	Shàoshāng	Shaoshang	Shōshō	소 상	So-Sang

N = Numbered system · Cc = Han Chinese characters · P = Pinyin Chinese
W = Wade-Giles Chinese · J = Japanese · Kc = Korean characters · K = Korean

F	G	R	V	L
Tchong-Fou	Mitte der Eingeweide	Чжун-фу	Trung-phū	Aula media
Iunn-Menn	Wolkentor	Юнь-мэнь	Van-môn	Porta nubium
Tienn-Fou	Himmelsbezirk	Тянь-фу	Thiên-phū	Aula caelestis
Sie-Po	Edle Helle	Ся-бай	Hiêp-bach	Candor coercitus
Tchre-Tsre	Ellenbogenteich	Чи-цзэ	Xich-trach	Lacus ulnaris
Krong-Tsoe	Äusserstes Loch	Кун-цзуй	Khóng-tôi	Extremitas cavi
Lie-Tsiue	Engpass	Ле-цюе	Liet-khuyét	Lacunae
Tsing-Tsiu	Abflusslauf	Цзин-цюй	Kinh-cu	Emissarium transitorium
Trae-Iuann	Grossquelle	Тай-юань	Thái-uyên	Vorago maior
Iu-Tsi	Daumenballengrenze	Юй-цзи	Ngu-té	Linea piscis
Chao-Chang	Geringer Handel	Шао-шан	Thiéu-thuong	Metallum structivum

F = French · G = German · R = Russian
V = Vietnamese · L = Latin

Large Intestine Meridian

N	Cc	P	W	J	Kc	K
X.1	商阳	Shāngyáng	Shangyang	Shōyō	상 양	Sang-Yang
X.2	二间	Èrjiān	Erhchien	Jikan	이 간	I-Gan
X.3	三间	Sānjiān	Sanchien	Sankan	삼 간	Sam-Gan
X.4	合谷	Hégǔ	Hoku	Gōkoku	합 곡	Hab-Gog
X.5	阳溪	Yángxī	Yangsi	Yōkei	양 계	Yang-Gye
X.6	偏历	Piānlì	Pienli	Henreki	편 력	Pyeon-Lyeog
X.7	温溜	Wēnliū	Wenliu	Onryū	온 유	On-yu
X.8	下廉	Xiàlián	Hsialien	Geren	하 렴	Ha-Ryeom
X.9	上廉	Shànglián	Shanglien	Jōren	상 렴	Sang-Ryeom
X.10	手三里	Shǒusānlǐ	Shousanli	Te no Sanri	수삼리	Su-Sam-Ri
X.11	曲池	Qūchi	Chuchih	Kyokuchi	곡 지	Gog-Ji
X.12	肘髎	Zhǒuliáo	Chouliao	Chūryō	주 료	Ju-Ryo
X.13	手五里	Wuli	Shouwuli	Te no Gori	수오리	Su-O-Ri
X.14	臂臑	Bìnào	Pinao	Hiju	비 노	Bi-No
X.15	肩髃	Jiānjú	Chienyu	Kengū	견 우	Gyeon-U
X.16	巨骨	Jùgǔ	Chuku	Kokotsu	거 골	Geo-Gol
X.17	天鼎	Tiāndǐng	Tienting	Tentei	천 정	Cheon-Jeong
X.18	扶突	[Neck] Fútu	Futu	Futotsu	부 돌	Bu-Dol
X.19	禾髎	[Nose] Heliao	Holiao	Karyō	(비)화료	Bi-Hwa-Ryo
X.20	迎香	Yingxiang	Yinghsiang	Geikō	영 향	Yeong-Hyang

N = Numbered system · Cc = Han Chinese characters · P = Pinyin Chinese
W = Wade-Giles Chinese · J = Japanese · Kc = Korean characters · K = Korean

F	G	R	V	L
Chang-Iang	Berater des Yang	Шан-ян	Thüóng-duong	Yang extremum
El-Tsienn	Zweites Fingerglied	Эр-цзянь	Nhi-gian	Interstitium alternum
Sann-Tsienn	Drittes Fingerglied	Сань-цзянь	Tam-gian	Interstitium tertium
Ro-Kou	Talbegegnung	Хэ-гу	Hiêp-cóc	Valles coniunctae
Iang-Tsri	Sonnenschlucht	Ян-си	Duong-khê	Rivulus yang
Pienn-Li	Seitliche Strecke	Пянь-ли	Thien-lich	Pervium obliquum
Oenn-Leou	Warmer Strom	Вэнь-лю	Ôn-lu	Amnis fovens
Sia-Lienn	Unterer Vorsprung des Armes	Ся-лянь	Ha-liêm	Angustiae inferae manus
Chang-Lienn	Oberer Vorsprung	Шан-лянь	Thuong-liem	Angustiae superae manus
Sann-Li	Drei Entfernungen	Шоу-сань-ли	Thú-tam-ly	Vicus tertius manus
Tsiou-Tchre	Gewundener Teich	Цюй-чи	Khúc-trì	Stagnum curvum
Tcheou-Tsiao	Grube des Ellenbogengelenkes	Чжоу-ляо	Trūu-giao	Cella cubiti
Ou-Li	Fünf Entfernungen	Шоу-у-ли	Ngũ-lý	Vicus quintus manus
Pi-Nao	Armmuskel	Би-нао	Tý-nhu	Latus lacerti
Tsienn-Iu	Schulterknochen	Цзянь-юй	Kiên-ngung	Promunturium humeri
Tsiu-Kou	Grossknochen-Schlüsselbein	Цзюй-гу	Cu-cöt	Os amplum
Tienn-Ting	Himmelsdreifuss	Тянь-дин	Thiên-danh	Tripus caelestis
Fou-Trou	Seitliche Vorwölbung	Фу-ту	Phò-dôt	Foramen aquaticum
Ro-Tsiao	Kornchengrube	Хэ-ляо	Hòa-giao	Cella frumentaria
Ing-Siang	Bewillkommnung des Duftes	Ин-сян	Nghinh-huong	Accipiens odores

F = French · G = German · R = Russian
V = Vietnamese · L = Latin

Stomach Meridian

N	Cc	P	W	J	Kc	K
XI.1	承泣	Chéngqì	Chengchi	Shōkyū	승 읍	Seung-Eub
XI.2	四白	Sibái	Szupai	Shihaku	사 백	Sa-Baeg
XI.3	巨髎	Jùliáo	Chuliao	Koryō	(면)거료	Myeon-Geo-Ryo
XI.4	地仓	Dìcāng	Titsang	Chisō	지 창	Ji-Chang
XI.5	大迎	Dàyíng	Taying	Daigei	대 영	Dae-Yeong
XI.6	颊车	Jiáchē	Chiache	Kyōsha	협 거	Hyeob-Geo
XI.7	下关	Xiàguān	Hsiakuan	Gekan	하 관	Ha-Gwan
XI.8	头维	Tóuwéi	Touwei	Zui	두 유	Du-Yu
XI.9	人迎	Rényíng	Jenying	Jingei	인 영	In-Yeong
XI.10	水突	Shuǐtū	Shuitu	Suitotsu	수 돌	Su-Doi
XI.11	气舍	Qìshè	Chishe	Kisha	기 사	Gi-sa
XI.12	缺盆	Quēpén	Chuehpen	Ketsubon	결 분	Gyeol-Bun
XI.13	气户	Qihù	Chihu	Kiko	기 호	Gi-Ho
XI.14	库房	Kùfáng	Kufang	Kobō	고 방	Go-Bang
XI.15	屋翳	Wūyi	Wuyi	Okuei	옥 예	Og-Ye
XI.16	膺窗	Yīnchuāng	Yingchuang	Yōsō	응 창	Eung-Chang
XI.17	乳中	Rǔzhōng	Juchung	Nyūchū	유 중	Yu-Jung
XI.18	乳根	Rǔgēn	Juken	Nyūkon	유 근	Yu-Geun
XI.19	不容	Bùróng	Puyung	Fuyō	불 용	Bul-Yong
XI.20	承满	Chéngmǎn	Chengman	Shōman	승 만	Seung-Man
XI.21	梁门	Liángmén	Liangmen	Ryōmon	양 문	Yang-Mun
XI.22	关门	Guānmén	Kuanmen	Kanmon	관 문	Gwan-Mun
XI.23	太乙	Tàiyǐ	Taiyi	Taiitsu	태 을	Tae-Eul

N = Numbered system · Cc = Han Chinese characters · P = Pinyin Chinese
W = Wade-Giles Chinese · J = Japanese · Kc = Korean characters · K = Korean

F	G	R	V	L
Treou-Oe	Kopfbindung	Чэн-ци	Däu-duy	Recipiens lacrimarum
Sia-Koann	Untere Grenze	Сы-бай	Ha-quan	Margo zygomaticus
Tsia-Tchre	Kieferknochen	Цзюй-ляо	Giáp-xa	Cella ampla
Tchreng-Tsri	Tränensammler	Ди-цан	Thua-kháp	Granarium terrestre
Se-Pae	Vierfache Helle	Да-ин	Tu-bach	Magnum accipiens
Tsiu-Tsiao	Grossgrube	Цзя-чэ	Cu-lieu	Maxilla
Ti-Tsrang	Erdspeicher	Ся-гуань	Dia-thuong	Clusa inferior
Ta-Ing	Grosse Bewillkommnung	Тоу-вэй	Dai-nghinh	Retinens capiti
Jenn-Ing	Menschenbewillkommnung	Жэнь-ин	Nhon-nghinh	Accipiens hominum
Choe-Trou	Wassersturz	Шуй-ту	Thũy-döt	Porta aquae
Tsri-Che	Atemhütte	Ци-шэ	Khi-xa	Domus ch'i
Tsiue-Prenn	Mangelschale	Цюе-пэнь	Khuyët-bön	Fossa supraclavicularis
Tsri-Rou	Atemtür	Ци-ху	Khi-hô	Ostium ch'i
Krou-Fang	Schatzhaus	Ку-фан	Khó-phong	Aerarium
Ou-I	Zimmerschirm	У-и	Oc-e	Tecti pluteus
Ing-Tchroang	Falkenfenster	Ин-чуан	Ung-song	Fenestra thoracis
Jou-Tchong	Brustmitte	Жу-чжун	Nhũ-trung	Medium mammae
Jou-Kenn	Brustwurzel	Жу-гэнь	Nhù-căn	Radix mammae
Pou-Jong	Ohne Inhalt	Бу-жун	Bat-dung	Non licet!
Tchreng-Mann	Aufnahme der Fülle	Чэн-мань	Thùa-mān	Recipiens plenitudinis
Leang-Menn	Balkentor	Лян-мэ̆нь	Luong-môn	Porta septi
Koann-Menn	Grenztor	Гуань-мэнь	Quang-mon	Porta clusae
Trae-I	Grosse Monade	Тай-и	Thai-āt	Unum maius

F = French · G = German · R = Russian
V = Vietnamese · L = Latin

N	Cc	P	W	J	Kc	K
XI.24	滑肉门	Huáròumén	Huajoumen	Katsunikumon	활육문	Hwal-Yug-Mun
XI.25	天枢	Tiānshū	Tienshu	Tensū	천 추	Cheon-Chu
XI.26	外陵	Wàilíng	Wailing	Gairyō	외 릉	Oe-Leung
XI.27	大巨	Dàjù	Tachu	Daiko	대 거	Dae-Geo
XI.28	水道	Shuǐdào	Shuitao	Suidō	수 도	Su-Do
XI.29	归来	Gūilái	Kueilai	Kirai	귀 래	Gwi-Rae
XI.30	气冲	Qìchōng	Chichung	Kishō	기 충	Gi-Chung
XI.31	髀关	Bìguān	Pikuan	Hikan	비 관	Bi-Gwan
XI.32	伏兔	[Femur] Fútū	Futu	Fukuto	복 토	Bog-To
XI.33	阴市	Yīnshì	Yinshih	Inshi	음 시	Eum-Si
XI.34	梁丘	Liángqiū	Liangchiu	Ryōkyū	양 구	Yang-Gu
XI.35	犊鼻	Dúbí	Tupi	Tokubi	독 비	Dog-Bi
XI.36	足三里	Zúsānlǐ	Tsusanli	Ashi no Sanri	족삼리	Jog-Sam-Ri
XI.37	上巨虚	Shàngjùxū	Shangchuhsu	Jōkokyo	(상거허)	Sang-Ryeom
XI.38	条口	Tiáokǒu	Tiaokou	Jōkō	조 구	Jo-Gu
XI.39	下巨虚	Xiàjùxū	Hsiachuhsu	Gekokyo	(하거허)	Ha-Ryeom
XI.40	丰隆	Fēnglóng	Fenglung	Hōryū	풍 륭	Pung-Lyung
XI.41	解溪	Jiěxī	Chiehhsi	Kaikei	해 계	Hae-Gye
XI.42	冲阳	Chōngyáng	Chungyang	Syōyō	충 양	Chung-Yang
XI.43	陷谷	Xiàngǔ	Hsienku	Kankoku	함 곡	Ham-Gog
XI.44	内庭	Nèitíng	Neiting	Naitei	내 정	Nae-eong
XI.45	厉兑	Lìdui	Litui	Reida	여 태	Yeo-Tae

N = Numbered system · Cc = Han Chinese characters · P = Pinyin Chinese
W = Wade-Giles Chinese · J = Japanese · Kc = Korean characters · K = Korean

F	G	R	V	L
Roa-Jeou	Glattes Fleisch	Хуа-жоу-мэнь	Huot-nhuc-mon	Porta carnis lubrica
Tienn-Tchrou	Himmelssäule	Тянь-шу	Thiĕn-xu	Cardo caeli
Oae-Ling	Aussenhügel	Вай-лин	Ngoai-lang	Tumulus externus
Ta-Tsiu	Grosse Macht	Да-цзюй	Dai-cu	Norma magna
Choe-Tao	Wasserweg	Шуй-дао	Thûy-dao	Via aquae
Koe-Lae	Rückkehr	Гуй-лай	Quy-lai	Vallis rivuli
Tsri-Tchrong	Atemstoss	Ци-чун	Khi-xung	Impedimentale ch'i
Pi-Koann	Schenkelgrenze	Би-гуань	Ty-quang	Clusa femoralis
Fou-Trou	Liegender Hase	Фу-ту	Phuc-thö	Lepus subreptus
Inn-Che	Schattenmarkt	Инь-ши	Âm-thi	Forum yin
Leang-Tsiou	Balkenhügel	Лян-цю	Luong-khuu	Monticulus septi
Tou-Pi	Kalbsnase	Ду-би	Dôc-tÿ	Nasus vituli
Sann-Li	Drei Entfernungen	Цзу-сань-ли	Túc-tam-lý	Vicus tertius pedis
Chang-Lienn	Oberer Vorsprung	Шан-цзюй-сюй	Thuong-cu-hu	Angustiae superiores aggeri ampli
Tiao-Kreou	Regelmässige Öffnung	Тяо-коу	Diéu-khàu	Os relaxationis
Sia-Lienn	Unterer Vorsprung	Ся-цзюй-сюй	Ha-cu-hu	Angustiae inferiores aggeri ampli
Fong-Long	Reiche Fulle	Фэн-лун	Phong-long	Abundantia
Tsie-Tsri	Tibiamulde	Цзе-си	Giäi-khé	Rivulus liberans
Tchrong-Iang	Yang-Angriff	Чун-ян	Xung-duong	Yang impedimentalis
Sienn-Kou	Versunkenes Tal	Сянь-гу	Ham-cöc	Vallis demersum
Nei-Ting	Innenhof	Нэй-тин	Noi-Dinh	Vestibulum internum
Li-Toe	Grausame Bezahlung	Ли-дуй	Lē-doai	Laetitia repressa

F = French · G = German · R = Russian
V = Vietnamese · L = Latin

Spleen Meridian

N	Cc	P	W	J	Kc	K
XII.1	隐白	Yinbai	Yinpai	Impaku	은 백	Eun-Baeg
XII.2	大都	Dàdū	Tatu	Daito	대 도	Dae-Do
XII.3	太白	Tàibái	Taipai	Taihaku	태 백	Tae-Baeg
XII.4	公孙	Gōngsūn	Kungsun	Kōson	공 손	Gong-Son
XII.5	商丘	Shāngqiū	Shangchiu	Shōkyū	상 구	Sang-Gu
XII.6	三阴交	Sānyīnjiāo	Sanyinchiao	Saninkō	삼음교	Sam-Eum-Gyo
XII.7	漏谷	Lòugŭ	Louku	Rōkoku	누 곡	Nu-Gog
XII.8	地机	Dìjī	Tichi	Chiki	지 기	Ji-Gi
XII.9	阴陵泉	Yīnlingquán	Yinlingchuan	Inryōsen	음릉천	Eum-Leung-Cheon
XII.10	血海	Xuèhǎi	Hsuehhai	Kekkai	혈 해	Hyeol-Hae
XII.11	箕门	Jīmén	Chimen	Kimon	기 문	Gag-Gi-Mun
XII.12	冲门	Chōngmén	Chongmen	Shōmon	충 문	Chung-Mun
XII.13	府舍	Fŭshè	Fushe	Fusha	부 사	Bu-Sa
XII.14	腹结	Fùjié	Fuchieh	Hukketsu	복 결	Bog-Gyeol
XII.15	大横	Dàhéng	Taheng	Daiō	대 횡	Dae-Hoeng
XII.16	腹哀	Fùāi	Fuai	Fukuai	복 애	Bog-Ae
XII.17	食窦	Shídòu	Shihtou	Shokutoku	식 두	Sig-Du
XII.18	天溪	Tiānxī	Tienhsi	Tenkei	천 계	Cheon-Gye
XII.19	胸乡	Xiōngxiāng	Hsiunghsiang	Kyōkyō	흉 향	Hyung-Hyang
XII.20	周荣	Zhōuróng	Chouyung	Shūei	주 영	Ju-Yeong
XII.21	大包	Dàbāo	Tapao	Daihō	대 포	Dae-Po

N = Numbered system · Cc = Han Chinese characters · P = Pinyin Chinese
W = Wade-Giles Chinese · J = Japanese · Kc = Korean characters · K = Korean

F	G	R	V	L
Inn-Po	Verborgene Helle	Инь-бай	An-bach	Candor occultus
Ta-Tou	Grosse Stadt	Да-ду	Dai-dô	Urbs magna
Trae-Po	Höchste Helle	Тай-бай	Thai-bach	Candidum maius
Kong-Soun	Fürstenenkel	Гун-сунь	Công-tôn	Caput metatarsalis hallucis
Chang-Tsiou	Beratungshügel	Шан-цю	Thuong-khuu	Monticulus tali
Sann-Inn-Tsiao	Treffpunkt der 3 Yin	Сань-инь-цзяо	Tam-ăm-giao	Copulatio trium yin
Leou-Kou	Offenes Tal	Лоу-гу	Lào-cŏc	Vallis percolationis
Ti-Tsi	Göttliche Kraft	Ди-цзи	Dia-co	Domus lienalis
Inn-Ling-Tsiuann	Hügelquelle	Инь-лин-цюань	Am-lăng-tuyèn	Fons tumuli yin
Siue-Rae	Blutmeer	Сюе-хай	Huyĕt-häi	Mare hsüeh
Tsi-Menn	Siebtor	Цзи-мэнь	Co-môn	Porta sagittarii
Tchrong-Menn	Angriffstor	Чун-мэнь	Xung-mon	Porta impedimentalis
Fou-Che	Bezirkshaus	Фу-шэ	Phū-xa	Domus aulicus
Fou-Tsie	Bauchnaht	Фу-цзе	Phúc-kiĕt	Nodus abdominalis
Ta-Rong	Grosskehre	Да-хэн	Phuc-ai	Transversum magnum
Fou-Ngae	Bauchleid	Фу-ай	Dai-hoành	Aegritudo abdominis
Che-Teou	Nahrungsöffnung	Ши-доу	Thuc-dôc	Clusa fortunae
Tienn-Tsri	Himmelsschlucht	Тянь-си	Thièn-khê	Rivulus caelestis
Siong-Siang	Brustbezirk	Сюн-сян	Hung-huong	Rus pectoris
Tcheou-Iong	Überall Glanz	Чжоу-жун	Châu-vinh	Castra angularis
Ta-Pao	Der grosse Entwickler	Да-бао	Dai-bào	Nexorium magnum lienalis

F = French · G = German · R = Russian
V = Vietnamese · L = Latin

Conception Vessel Meridian

N	Cc	P	W	J	Kc	K
XIII.1	会阴	Huìyīn	Huiyin	Ein	회 음	Hoe-Eum
XIII.2	曲骨	Qūgǔ	Chuku	Kyokkotsu	곡 골	Gog-Gol
XIII.3	中极	Zhōngjí	Chungchi	Chūkyoku	중 극	Jung-Geug
XIII.4	关元	Guānyuán	Kuanyuan	Kangen	관 원	Gwan-Weon
XIII.5	石门	Shímén	Shihmen	Sekimon	석 문	Seog-Mun
XIII.6	气海	Qìhǎi	Chihai	Kikai	기 해	Gi-Hae
XIII.7	阴交	[Abdomen] Yīnjiāo	Yinchiao	Inkō	음 교	Eum-Gyo
XIII.8	神阙	Shénquè	Shenchueh	Shinketsu	신 궐	Sin-Gweol
XIII.9	水分	Shuǐfēn	Shuifen	Suibun	수 분	Su-Bun
XIII.10	下脘	Xiàwǎn	Hsiawan	Gekan	하 완	Ha-Wan
XIII.11	建里	Jiànlí	Chienli	Kenri	건 리	Geon-Ri
XIII.12	中脘	Zhōngwǎn	Chungwan	Chūkan	중 완	Jung-Wan
XIII.13	上脘	Shàngwǎn	Shanwan	Jōkan	상 완	Sang-Wan
XIII.14	巨阙	Jùquè	Chuchueh	Koketsu	거 궐	Geo-Gweol
XIII.15	鸠尾	Jiūwěi	Chiuwei	Kyūbi	구 미	Gu-Mi
XIII.16	中庭	Zhōngtíng	Chungting	Chūtei	중 정	Jung-Jeong
XIII.17	膻中	Shānzhōng	Shanchung	Danchū	전 중	Jeon-Jung
XIII.18	玉堂	Yùtáng	Yutang	Gyokudō	옥 당	Og-Dang
XIII.19	紫宫	[Chest] Zigōng	Tzukung	Shikyū	자 궁	Ja-Gung
XIII.20	华盖	Huágài	Huakai	Kagai	화 개	Hwa-Gae
XIII.21	璇玑	Xuánjī	Hsuanchi	Senki	선 기	Seon-Gi
XIII.22	天突	Tiāntū	Tientu	Tentotsu	천 돌	Cheon-Dol
XIII.23	廉泉	Liánquán	Lienchuan	Rensen	염 천	Yeom-Cheon
XIII.24	承浆	Chéngjiāng	Chengchiang	Shōshō	승 장	Seung-Jahg

N = Numbered system · Cc = Han Chinese characters · P = Pinyin Chinese
W = Wade-Giles Chinese · J = Japanese · Kc = Korean characters · K = Korean

F	G	R	V	L
Roe-Inn	Geschlectspunkt	Хуэй-инь	Hôi-âm	Yin conventi
Tsiou-Kou	Gebogener Knochen	Цюй-гу	Khúc-cốt	Os curvum
Tchong-Tsi	Mittlerer Gipfelpunkt	Чжун-цзи	Trung-cuc	Conquisitorium vesicale
Koann-Iuann	Grenz-Vorsprung	Гуань-юань	Quang-nguyên	Prima clusarum
Che-Menn	Stein-Tor	Ши-мэнь	Thach-môn	Porta lapidea
Tsri-Rae	Meer der Energie	Ци-хай	Khi-hāi	Mare ch'i
Inn-Tsiao	Yin-Vereinigung	Инь-цзяо	Ām-giao	Copulatio yin
Chenn-Koann	Gottliche Grenze	Шэнь-цюе	Than-khuyět	Medium umbilici
Choe-Fenn	Wasserverteilung	Шуй-фэнь	Thùý-phăn	Aquae divisae
Sia-Koann	Unterer Kanal	Ся-вань	Ha-uyēn	Foramen pyloricum
Tsienn-Li	Die niedergelassene Ortschaft	Цзянь-ли	Kien-ly	Vicus constitutus
Tchong-Koann	Mittlerer Kanal	Чжун-вань	Trung-uyen	Conquisitorium stomachi
Chang-Koann	Oberer Kanal	Шан-вань	Thuong-uyen	Foramen cardiacum
Tsiu-Koann	Macht-Grenze	Цзюй-цюе	Cu-khuyet	Conquisitorium cardiale
Tsiou-Oe	Tauben-Schwanz	Цзю-вэй	Cuu-ӱy	Cauda columbina
Tchong-Ting	Mittlerer Hof	Чжун-тин	Trung-dinh	Vestibulum medium
Trann-Tchong	Brustmitte	Тань-чжун	Chiên-trung	Atrium pectoris
Iu-Trang	Jade-Halle	Юй-тан	Ngoc-duong	Atrium iaspidis
Tsre-Kong	Purpur-Palast	Цзы-гун	Tü-cuug	Conclave purpureum
Roa-Kae	Blumen-Decke	Хуа-гай	Hoa-cai	Tegmen floreum
Siuann-Tsi	Jade-Perle	Сюань-цзи	Triën-co	Dioptra mobilis
Tienn-Trou	Himmels-Pfad	Тянь-ту	Thien-dot	Processus caelestis
Lienn-Tsiuann	Seitliche Quelle	Лянь-цюань	Liêm-tuyën	Fons in angustiis
Tchreng-Tsiang	Flüssigkeitsaufnahme	Чэн-цзян	Thùa-tuong	Recipiens liquoris

F = French · G = German · R = Russian
V = Vietnamese · L = Latin

Governor Vessel Meridian

N	Cc	P	W	J	Kc	K
XIV.1	长强	Chángqiáng	Changchiang	Chōkyō	장 강	Jang-Gang
XIV.2	腰俞	Yāoshū	Yaoshu	Yōyu	요 수	Yo-Su
XIV.3	腰阳关	Yāoyángguān	Yao Yangkuan	Koshi no Yōkan	요양관	Yo-Yang-Gwan
XIV.4	命门	Mìngmén	Mingmen	Meimon	명 문	Myeong-Mun
XIV.5	悬枢	Xuánshū	Hsuanshu	Kensū	현 추	Hyeon-Chu
XIV.6	脊中	Jìzhōng	Chichung	Sekichū	척 중	Cheog-Jung
XIV.7	中枢	Zhōngshū	Chungshu	Chūsū	중 추	Jung-Chu
XIV.8	筋缩	Jīnsuō	Chinso	Kinshuku	근 축	Geung-Chug
XIV.9	至阳	Zhìyáng	Chihyang	Shiyō	지 양	Ji-Yang
XIV.10	灵台	Língtái	Lingtai	Reidai	영 대	Yeong-Dae
XIV.11	神道	Shéndào	Shentao	Shindō	신 도	Sin-Do
XIV.12	身柱	Shēnzhù	Shenchu	Shinchū	신 주	Sin-Ju
XIV.13	陶道	Táodào	Taotao	Tōdō	도 도	Do-Do
XIV.14	大椎	Dázhuī	Tachui	Daitsui	대 퇴	Dae-Toe
XIV.15	哑门	Yămén	Yamen	Amon	아 문	A-Mun
XIV.16	风府	Fengfŭ	Fengfu	Fūfu	풍 부	Pung-Bu
XIV.17	脑户	Năohù	Naohu	Nōko	뇌 호	Noe-Ho
XIV.18	强间	Qiángjiān	Chiangchien	Kyōkan	강 간	Gang-Gan
XIV.19	后顶	Hòudĭng	Houting	Gochō	후 정	Hu-Jeong
XIV.20	百会	Băihuì	Paihui	Hyakue	백 회	Baeg-Hoe
XIV.21	前顶	Qiándĭng	Chienting	Zenchō	전 정	Jeon-Jeong
XIV.22	囟会	Xìnhuì	Hsinhui	Shine	신 회	Sin-Hoe
XIV.23	上星	Shàngxīng	Shanghsing	Jōsei	상 성	Sang-Seong
XIV.24	神庭	Shéntíng	Shenting	Shintei	신 정	Sin-Jeong
XIV.25	素髎	Sùliáo	Suliao	Soryō	소 료	So-Ryo
XIV.26	人中	Rénzhōng	Jenchung	Suikō	수 구	Su-Gu
XIV.27	兑端	Duìduān	Tuituan	Datan	태 단	Tae-Dan
XIV.28	龈交	Yínjiāo	Yinchiao	Ginkō	은 교	Eun-Gyo

N = Numbered system · Cc = Han Chinese characters · P = Pinyin Chinese
W = Wade-Giles Chinese · J = Japanese · Kc = Korean characters · K = Korean

F	G	R	V	L
Tchrang-Tsiang	Wachsen der Kraft	Чан-цян	Truong-cuòng	Incrementum et vigor
Iao-Iu	Zustimmungspunkt der Lumbalregion	Яо-шу	Yêu-du	Inductorium lumbale
Iang-Koann	Yang-Grenze	Ян-гуань	Duong-quang	Clusa yang regentis
Ming-Menn	Lebenstor	Мин-мэнь	Mang-mon	Porta fortunae
Siuann-Tchrou	Hängender Pfeiler	Сюань-шу	Huyēn-xu	Cardo suspensus
Tsi-Tchong	Mittle der Wirbelsäule	Цзи-чжун	Tich-trung	Medium spinae
Tchong-Tchrou	* All numbers after 7 are advanced by one.	Чжун-шу		Cardo medius
Tsinn-Chou	Muskelstraffer	Цзинь-со	Cân-suc	Nervi constricti
Tche-Iang	Ankunft des Yang	Чжи-ян	Chi-duong	Yang supremus
Ling-Trae	Geisterterrasse	Лин-тай	Linh-dai	Turris responsiva
Chenn-Tao	Göttlicher Weg	Шэнь-дао	Thān-dao	Via shen
Chenn-Tchou	Körpersäule	Шэнь-чжу	Than-tru	Columna personae
Trao-Tao	Wandlungsweg	Тао-дао	Dao-dao	Via figulina
Pae-Lao	Hundert Mühen	Да-чжуй	Dai-chuy	Omnium defatigationum
Ia-Menn	Tor des Schweigens	Я-мэнь	Â-môn	Porta infantiae
Fong-Fou	Windbezirk	Фэн-фу	Phong-phu	Aula venti
Nao-Rou	Gehirntür	Нао-ху	Näo-hö	Ostium cerebri
Tsiang-Tsienn	Ort der Kraft	Цян-цзянь	Cuòng-gian	Interstitium vigoris
Reou-Ting	Hinterer Kopfhügel	Хоу-дин	Hâu-dánh	Parietale posterius
Pae-Roe	Der hundertfache Sammler	Бай-хуэй	Bách-höi	Conventus omnium
Tsienn-Ting	Vorderer Hügel	Цянь-дин	Tiën-dānh	Parietale anterius
Tchroang-Roe	Schädeldeckenpult	Син-хуэй	Tinh-hôi	Fonticulus maior
Chang-Sing	Oberer Stern	Шан-син	Thuong-tinh	Stella superior
Chenn-Ting	Göttlicher Hof	Шэнь-тин	Thān-dinh	Vestibulum shen
Sou-Tsiao	Das einfache Loch	Су-ляо	To-lieu	Rex faciei
Choe-Keou	Wassergraben	Жэнь-чжун	Thuy-cău	Canalis aquae
Toe-Toann	Oberer Lippenrand	Дуй-дуань	Doài-doan	Promuntorium laetitiae
Inn-Tsiao	Zahnfleischpunkt	Инь-цзяо	Ngân-giao	Copulatio gingivalis

F = French · G = German · R = Russian
V = Vietnamese · L = Latin

PINYIN
CHINESE
ALPHABETIZED

P	J	F	Ns	
Baihuanshu	Hakkanyu	Pae-Roann-Iu	BL	30
Baihui	Hyakue	Pae-Roe	GV	20
Baohuang	Hoko	Pae-Roang	BL	48/43
Benshen	Honshin	Penn-Chenn	GB	13
Biguan	Hikan	Pi-Koann	ST	31
Binao	Hiju	Pi-Nao	LI	14
Bingfeng	Heifu	Tchreng-Fong	SI	12
Bulang	Horo	Pou-Lang	K	22
Burong	Fuyo	Pou-Jong	ST	19
Changqiang	Chokyo	Tchrang-Tsiang	GV	1
Chengfu	Shofo	Tchreng-Fou	BL	50/36
Chengguang	Gosho	Ou-Tchrong	BL	6
Chengjiang	Shosho	Tchreng-Tsiang	CV	24
Chengjin	Shokin	Tchreng-Tsinn	BL	56
Chengling	Shorei	Tcheng-Ling	GB	18
Chengman	Shoman	Tchreng-Mann	ST	20
Chengqi	Shokyu	Treou-Oe	ST	1
Chengshan	Shozan	Tchreng-Chann	BL	57
Chize	Shakutaku	Tchre-Tsre	LU	5
Chongmen	Shomon	Tchrong-Menn	SP	12
Chongyang	Syoyo	Fong-Long	ST	42
Ciliao	Jiryo	Tsre-Tsiao	BL	32
Dabao	Daiho	Ta-Pao	SP	21
Dachangshu	Daichoyu	Ta-Tchrang-Iu	BL	25
Dadu	Taihaku	Trae-Po	SP	3
Dadun	Daiton	Ta-Toun	LV	1

P = Pinyin Chinese · J = Japanese
F = French · Ns = Numbered system

P	J	F	Ns	
Dahe	Daikaku	Ta-Ro	K	12
Daheng	Dato	Ta-Rong	SP	15
Daimai	Suiko	Choe-Keou	GB	26
Daju	Daiko	Ta-Tsiu	ST	27
Daling	Dairyo	Ta-Ling	CS	7
Danshu	Tanyu	Tann-Iu	BL	19
Dashu	Daijo	Ta-Tchrou	BL	11
Daying	Daigei	Se-Pae	ST	5
Dazhong	Daisho	Ta-Tchong	K	4
Dazhui	Daitsui	Pae-Lao	GV	14
Dicang	Chiso	Tohreng-Tsri	ST	4
Diji	Chiki	Ti-Tsi	SP	8
Diwuhui	Chigoe	Ti-Ou-Roe	GB	42
Dubi	Tokubi	Tou-Pi	ST	35
Duiduan	Datan	Toe-Toann	GV	27
Dushu	Tokuyu	Tou-Iu	BL	16
Erjian	Jikan	El-Tsienn	LI	2
Ermen	Jimon	Se-Tchoe-Kong	TH	21
Feishu	Haiyu	Fei-Iu	BL	13
Feiyang	Hiyo	Fei-Iang	BL	58
Fengchi	Fuchi	Fong-Tchre	GB	20
Fengfu	Fufu	Fong-Fou	GV	16
Fenglong	Horyu	Fong-Long	ST	40
Fengmen	Fumon	Fong-Menn	BL	12
Fengshi	Fushi	Fong-Che	GB	31
Fuai	Fukai	Fou-Ngae	SP	16

P = Pinyin Chinese · J = Japanese
F = French · Ns = Numbered system

P	J	F	Ns
Fubai	Fuhaku	Feou-Pae	GB 10
Fufen	Fubun	Fou-Fenn	BL 36/41
Fujie	Hukketsu	Fou-Tsie	SP 14
Fuliu	Fukuryu	Fou-Leou	K 7
Fushe	Fusha	Fou-Che	SP 13
Futu	Fukuto	Fou-Trou	ST 32
Futu	Futotsu	Fou-Trou	LI 18
Fuxi	Fugeki	Feou-Tsri	BL 52/38
Fuyang	Fuyo	Fou-Iang	BL 59
Ganshu	Kanyu	Kann-Iu	BL 18
Gaohuang	Koko	Kao-Roang	BL 38/43
Geguan	Kakkan	Ko-Koann	BL 41/46
Geshu	Kakuyu	Ko-Iu	BL 17
Gongsun	Koson	Kong-Soun	SP 4
Guanchong	Kansyo	Koann-Tchrong	TH 1
Guangming	Komei	Koang-Ming	GB 37
Guanmen	Kanmon	Koann-Menn	ST 22
Guanyuan	Kangen	Koann-Iuann	CV 4
Guanyuanshu	Kangenyu	Koann-Iuann-Iu	BL 26
Guilai	Kirai	Koe-Iae	ST 29
Hanyan	Ganen	Rann-Ia	GB 4
Hegu	Gokoku	Ro-Kou	LI 4
Heliao	Karyo	Ro-Tsiao	LI 19
Heliao	Waryo	Ro-Tsiao	TH 22
Henggu	Okotsu	Rong-Kou	K 11
Heyang	Goyo	Ro-Iang	BL 55
Houding	Gocho	Reou-Ting	GV 19

P = Pinyin Chinese · J = Japanese
F = French · Ns = Numbered system

P	J	F	Ns
Houxi	Gokei	Reou Tsri	SI 3
Huagai	Kagai	Roa-Kae	CV 20
Huangmen	Komon	Roang-Menn	BL 46/51
Huangshu	Koyu	Roang-Iu	K 16
Huantiao	Kancho	Roann-Tsiao	GB 30
Huaroumen	Katsunikumon	Roa-Jeou	ST 24
Huiyang	Eyo	Roe-Iang	BL 35
Huiyin	Ein	Roe-Inn	CV 1
Huizong	Eso	Roe-Tsong	TH 7
Hunmen	Konmon	Roun-Menn	BL 42/47
Jiache	Kyosha	Tsiu-Tsri	ST 6
Jianjing	Kensei	Tienn-Tsing	GB 21
Jianju	Kengu	Tsienn-Iu	LI 15
Jianli	Kenri	Tsienn-Li	CV 11
Jianliao	Kenryo	Tsienn-Tsiao	TH 14
Jianshi	Kanshi	Tsienn-Che	CS 5
Jianwaishu	Kengaiyu	Tsienn Oae	SI 14
Jianzhen	Kenei	Tsienn Tchenn	SI 9
Jianzhongshu	Kenchuyu	Tsienn Tchong	SI 15
Jiaosun	Kakuson	Tsio-Soun	TH 20
Jiaoxin	Koshin	Tsiao-Sinn	K 8
Jiexi	Kaikei	Tsie-Tsri	ST 41
Jimai	Kyumyaku	Tsiou-Tsiuann	LV 12
Jimen	Kimon	Tsi-Menn	SP 11
Jinggu	Keikotsu	Tsing-Kou	BL 64
Jingmen	Keimon	Tsing-Menn	GB 25

P = Pinyin Chinese · J = Japanese
F = French · Ns = Numbered system

P	J	F	Ns
Jingming	Seimei	Tsing-Ming	BL 1
Jingqu	Keikyo	Tsing-Tsiu	LU 8
Jinmen	Kinmon	Tsinn-Menn	BL 63
Jinsuo	Kinshuku	Tsinn-Chou	GV 8
Jiquan	Kyokusen	Tsi Tsiuann	HT 1
Jiuwei	Kyubi	Tsiou-Oe	CV 15
Jizhong	Sekichu	Tsi-Tchong	GV 6
Jueyinshu	Ketsuinyu	Tsiue-Inn-Iu	BL 14
Jugu	Kokotsu	Tsiu-Kou	LI 16
Juliao	Koryo	Tsia-Tchre	ST 3
Juliao	Kyoryo	Tsiu-Tsiao	GB 29
Juque	Koketsu	Tsiu-Koann	CV 14
Kongzui	Kosai	Krong-Tsoe	LU 6
Kufang	Kobo	Krou-Fang	ST 14
Kunlun	Konron	Kroun-Loun	BL 60
Laogong	Rokyu	Lao-Kong	CS 8
Liangmen	Ryomon	Leang-Menn	ST 21
Liangqiu	Ryokyu	Leang-Tsiou	ST 34
Lianquan	Rensen	Lienn-Tsiuann	CV 23
Lidui	Reida	Li-Toe	ST 45
Lieque	Rekketsu	Lie-Tsiue	LU 7
Ligou	Reiko	Li-Keou	LV 5
Lingdao	Kyokusen	Tsi-Tsiuann	HT 4
Lingtai	Reidai	Ling-Trae	GV 10
Lingxu	Reikyo	Ling-Siu	K 24
Linqi	Atama no Rinkyu	Linn-Tsri	GB 15
Linqi	Ashi no Rinkyu	Linn-Tsri	GB 41

P = Pinyin Chinese · J = Japanese
F = French · Ns = Numbered system

P	J	F	Ns	
Lougu	Rokoku	Leou-Kou	SP	7
Luoque	Rakkyaku	Lo-Tsri	BL	8
Luxi	Rosoku	Lou-Si	TH	19
Meichong	Bisho	Mei-Tchrong	BL	3
Mingmen	Meimon	Ming-Menn	GV	4
Muchuang	Mokuso	Mou-Tchroan	GB	16
Naohu	Noko	Nao-Rou	GV	17
Naohui	Jue	Nao-Roe	TH	13
Naokong	Noku	Nao-Krong	GB	19
Naoshu	Juyu	Nao-Iu	SI	10
Neiguan	Naikan	Nei-Koann	CS	6
Neiting	Naitei	Nei-Ting	ST	44
Pangguangshu	Bokoyu	Prang-Koang-Iu	BL	28
Pianli	Henreki	Pienn-Li	LI	6
Pishu	Hiyu	Pi-Iu	BL	20
Pohu	Hakko	Pro-Rou	BL	37/42
Pushen	Bokushin	Prou-Chenn	BL	61
Qianding	Zencho	Tsienn-Ting	GV	21
Qiangjian	Kyokan	Tsiang-Tsienn	GV	18
Qiangu	Zenkoku	Tsienn-Kou	SI	2
Qiaoyin	Atama no Kyōin	Tsiao-Inn	GB	11
Qichong	Kisho	Tsri-Tchrong	ST	30
Qihai	Kikai	Tsri-Rae	CV	6
Qihaishu	Kikaiyu	Tsri-Rae-Iu	BL	24
Qihu	Kiko	Tsri-Roe	ST	13
Qimai	Keimyaku	Tchre-Mo	TH	18

P = Pinyin Chinese · J = Japanese
F = French · Ns = Numbered system

P	J	F	Ns	
Qimen	Kimon	Tsri-Menn	LV	14
Qinglengyuan	Seireien	Tsring-Ling-Iuann	TH	11
Qingling	Seirei	Tsring-Ling	HT	2
Qishe	Kisha	Tsri-Che	ST	11
Qiuxu	Kyukyo	Tsiou-Siu	GB	40
Qixue	Kiketsu	Tsri-Tsiue	KI	13
Quanliao	Kenryo	Tsiuann Tsiao	SI	18
Qubin	Kyokubin	Tsiou-Ping	GB	7
Quchai	Kyokusa	Tsiou-Tchrea	BL	4
Quchi	Kyokuchi	Tsiou-Tchre	LI	11
Quepen	Ketsubon	Tsiue-Prenn	ST	12
Qugu	Kyokotsu	Tsiou-Kou	CV	2
Ququan	Kyokusen	Tsiou-Tsiuann	LV	8
Quyuan	Kyokuen	Tsiou Iuann	SI	13
Quze	Kyokutaku	Tsiou-Tsre	CS	3
Rangu	Yusen	Iong-Tsiuann	KI	2
Renying	Jingei	Jenn-Ing	ST	9
Renzhong	Suiko	Choe-Keou	GV	26
Riyue	Jitsugetsu	Je-Iue	GB	24
Rugen	Nyukon	Jou-Kenn	ST	18
Ruzhong	Nyuchu	Jou-Tchroang	ST	17
Sanjian	Sankan	Sann-Tsienn	LI	3
Sanjiaoshu	Sanshoyu	Sann-Tsiao-Iu	BL	22
Sanyangluo	Sanyoraku	Sann-Iang-Lo	TH	8
Sanyinjiao	Saninko	Sann-Inn-Tsiao	SP	6
Shangguan	Kakushujin	Kro-Tchou-Jenn	GB	3

P = Pinyin Chinese · J = Japanese
F = French · Ns = Numbered system

P	J	F	Ns	
Shangjuxu	Jokoyo	Chang-Lienn	ST	37
Shanglian	Joren	Chang-Lienn	LI	9
Shangliao	Joryo	Chang-Tsiao	BL	31
Shangqiu	Shokyu	Chang-Tsiou	SP	5
Shangqu	Shokyoku	Chang-Tsiou	KI	17
Shangwan	Jokan	Chang-Koann	CV	13
Shangxing	Josei	Chang-Sing	GV	23
Shangyang	Shoyo	Chang-Iang	LI	1
Shanzhong	Danchu	Trann-Tchong	CV	17
Shaochong	Shosho	Chao-Tsrong	HT	9
Shaofu	Shofu	Chao Fou	HT	8
Shaohai	Shokai	Chao Rae	HT	3
Shaoshang	Shosho	Chao-Chang	LU	11
Shaoze	Shaotaku	Chao Tsre	SI	1
Shencang	Shinzo	Chenn-Tsrang	KI	25
Shendao	Shindo	Chenn-Tao	GV	11
Shenfeng	Shimpo	Chenn-Fong	KI	23
Shenmai	Shinmyaku	Chenn-Mo	BL	62
Shenmen	Shinmon	Chenn-Menn	HT	7
Shenque	Shinketsu	Chenn-Koann	CV	8
Shenshu	Jinyu	Chenn-Iu	BL	23
Shentang	Shindo	Chenn-Trang	BL	39/44
Shenting	Shintei	Chenn-Ting	GV	24
Shenzhu	Shinchu	Chenn-Tchrou	GV	12
Shidou	Shoktoku	Che-Teou	SP	17
Shiquan	Sekikan	Che-Koann	KI	18

P = Pinyin Chinese · J = Japanese
F = French · Ns = Numbered system

P	J	F	Ns	
Shimen	Sekimon	Che-Menn	CV	5
Shousanli	Te no Sanri	Sann-Li	LI	10
Shuaigu	Sokkoku	Choae-Kou	GB	8
Shufu	Yufu	Iu-Fou	KI	27
Shugu	Ashi no Tsukoku	Trong-Kou	BL	65
Shuidao	Suido	Choe-Tao	ST	28
Shuifen	Suibun	Choe-Fenn	CV	9
Shuiquan	Suisen	Choe-Tsiuann	KI	5
Shuitu	Suitotsu	Choe-Trou	ST	10
Sibai	Shihaku	Sia-Koann	ST	2
Sidu	Shitoku	Se-Tou	TH	9
Siman	Shiman	Se-Mann	KI	14
Sizhukong	Shichikuku	El-Menn	TH	23
Suliao	Soryo	Sou-Tsiao	GV	25
Taibai	Taihaku	Trae-Po	SP	3
Taichong	Taisho	Trae-Tsienn	LV	3
Taixi	Taikei	Trae-Tsri	KI	3
Taiyi	Taiitsu	Trae-I	ST	23
Taiyuan	Taien	Trae-Iuann	LU	9
Taodao	Todo	Trao-Tao	GV	13
Tianchi	Tenchi	Tienn-Tchre	CS	1
Tianchong	Tensho	Tienn-Tchrong	GB	9
Tianchuang	Tenso	Tsienn-Tchroang	SI	16
Tianding	Tentei	Tienn-Iu	LI	17
Tianfu	Tempu	Tienn-Fou	LU	3
Tianjing	Tensei	Tienn-Tsing	TH	10

P = Pinyin Chinese · J = Japanese
F = French · Ns = Numbered system

P	J	F	Ns
Tianliao	Tenryo	Tsienn-Tsiao	TH 15
Tianquan	Tensen	Tienn-Tsiuann	CS 2
Tianrong	Tenyo	Tiann-Jong	SI 17
Tianshu	Tensu	Tienn-Tchrou	ST 25
Tiantu	Tentotsu	Tienn-Trou	CV 22
Tianxi	Tenkei	Tienn-Tsri	SP 18
Tianyou	Tenyu	Tienn-Iou	TH 16
Tianzhu	Tenchu	Tienn-Tchou	BL 10
Tianzong	Tenso	Tienn-Tsong	SI 11
Tiaokou	Joko	Tiao-Kreou	ST 38
Tinggong	Choyu	Ting Kong	SI 19
Tinghui	Choe	Ting-Roe	GB 2
Tonggu	Ashi no Tsukoku	Trong-Kou	BL 66
Tonggu	Hara no Tsukoku	Trong-Kou	KI 20
Tongli	Tsuri	Trong Li	HT 5
Tongtian	Tsuten	Trong-Tienn	BL 7
Tongziliao	Doshiryo	Trong-Tse-Tsiao	GB 1
Touwei	Zui	Ta-Ing	ST 8
Waiguan	Gaikan	Oae-Koann	TH 5
Wailing	Gairyo	Oae-Ling	ST 26
Waiqiu	Gaikyu	Oae-Tsiou	GB 36
Wangu	Wankotsu	Oann-Kou	SI 4
Wangu	Kankotsu	Oann-Kou	GB 12
Weicang	Iso	Oe-Tsrang	BL 45/50
Weidao	Ido	Oe-Tao	GB 28
Weishu	Iyu	Oe-Iu	BL 21

P = Pinyin Chinese · J = Japanese
F = French · Ns = Numbered system

P	J	F	Ns	
Weiyang	Iyo	Oe-Iang	BL	53/39
Weizhong	Ichu	Oe-Tchong	BL	54/40
Wenliu	Onryu	Oenn-Leou	LI	7
Wuchu	Gosho	Ou-Tchrou	BL	5
Wuli	Te no Gori	Ou-Li	LI	13
Wuli	Ashi no Gori	Ou-Li	LV	10
Wushu	Gosu	Ou-Tchrou	GB	27
Wuyi	Okuei	Ou-I	ST	15
Xiabai	Kyohaku	Sie-Po	LU	4
Xiaguan	Gekan	Ti-Tsrang	ST	7
Xiajuxu	Gekokyo	Sia-Lienn	ST	39
Xialian	Geren	Sia-Lienn	LI	8
Xialiao	Geryo	Sia-Tsiao	BL	34
Xiangu	Kankoku	Sienn-Kou	ST	43
Xiaochangshu	Shochoyu	Siao-Tchrang-Iu	BL	27
Xiaohai	Shokai	Siao-Rae	SI	8
Xiaoluo	Shoreki	Siao-Io	TH	12
Xiawan	Gekan	Sia-Koann	CV	10
Xiaxi	Kyokei	Sie-Tsri	GB	43
Xiguan	Shitsukan	Si-Koann	LV	7
Ximen	Gekimon	Tsri-Menn	CS	4
Xingjian	Daiton	Ta-Toun	LV	2
Xinhui	Shine	Tchroang-Roe	GV	22
Xinshu	Shinyu	Sinn-Iu	BL	15
Xiongxiang	Kyokyo	Siong-Siang	SP	19
Xiyangguan	Ashi no Yokan	Iang-Koann	GB	33

P = Pinyin Chinese · J = Japanese
F = French · Ns = Numbered system

P	J	F	Ns	
Xuanji	Senki	Siuann-Tsi	CV	21
Xuanli	Kenri	Siuann-Iou	GB	6
Xuanlu	Kenro	Siuann-Lou	GB	5
Xuanshu	Kensu	Siuann-Tchrou	GV	5
Xuanzhong	Kensho	Siuann-Tchrong	GB	39
Xuehai	Kekkai	Siue-Rae	SP	10
Yamen	Amon	Ia-Menn	GV	15
Yangbai	Yohaku	Iang-Pae	GB	14
Yangchi	Yochi	Iang-Tchre	TH	4
Yangfu	Yoho	Iang-Fou	GB	38
Yanggang	Yoko	Iang-Kang	BL	43/48
Yanggu	Yokoku	Iang-Kou	SI	5
Yangjiao	Yoko	Iang-Tsiou	GB	35
Yanglao	Yoro	Iang-Lao	SI	6
Yanglingquan	Yoryosen	Iang-Ling-Tsiuann	GB	34
Yangxi	Yokei	Iang-Tsri	LI	5
Yaoshu	Yoyu	Iao-Iu	GV	2
Yaoyangguan	Koshi no Yokan	Iang-Koann	GV	3
Yemen	Ekimon	Ie-Menn	TH	2
Yifeng	Eifu	I-Fong	TH	17
Yinbai	Impaku	In-Po	SP	1
Yinbao	Impo	Inn-Pao	LV	9
Yindu	Into	Inn-Tou	KI	19
Yingchuang	Yoso	Ing-Tchroang	ST	16
Yingu	Inkoku	Inn-Kou	KI	10
Yingxiang	Geiko	Ing-Siang	LI	20

P = Pinyin Chinese · J = Japanese
F = French · Ns = Numbered system

P	J	F	Ns
Yinjiao	Ginko	Inn-Tsiao	GV 28
Yinjiao	Inko	Inn-Tsiao	CV 7
Yinlian	Inren	Inn-Lienn	LV 11
Yinlingquan	Inryosen	Inn-Ling-Tsiuann	SP 9
Yinmen	Inmon	Inn-Menn	BL 51/37
Yinshi	Inshi	Inn-Che	ST 33
Yinxi	Ingeki	Inn Tsri	HT 6
Yishe	Isha	I-Che	BL 44/49
Yixi	Iki	I-Si	BL 40/45
Yongquan	Yusen	Iong-Tsiuann	KI 1
Youmen	Yufu	Iu-Fou	KI 27
Yuanye	Eneki	Iuann-Ie	GB 22
Yuji	Gyosai	Iu-Tsi	LU 10
Yunmen	Unmon	Iunn-Menn	LU 2
Yutang	Gyokudo	Iu-Trang	CV 18
Yuzhen	Gyokuchin	Iu-Tchenn	BL 9
Yuzhong	Wakuchu	Rouo-Tchrong	KI 26
Zanzhu	Sanchiku	Tsroann-Tchrou	BL 2
Zhangmen	Shomon	Tchang-Menn	LV 13
Zhaohai	Shokai	Tchao-Rae	KI 6
Zhejin	Chokin	Tchre-Tsinn	GB 23
Zhengying	Shoei	Tcheng-Ing	GB 17
Zhibian	Chippen	Tche-Pienn	BL 49/54
Zhigou	Shiko	Tche-Keou	TH 6

P = Pinyin Chinese · J = Japanese
F = French · Ns = Numbered system

P	J	F	Ns	
Zhishi	Shishitsu	Tche-Che	BL	47/52
Zhiyang	Shiyo	Tche-Iang	GV	9
Zhiyin	Shiin	Tche-Inn	BL	67
Zhizheng	Shisei	Tche-Tcheng	SI	7
Zhongchong	Chusho	Tchong-Tchrong	CS	9
Zhongdu	Chuto	Tchong-Fong	LV	6
Zhongdu	Chutoku	Sia-Tou	GB	32
Zhongfeng	Chuho	Tchong-Fong	LV	4
Zhongfu	Chufu	Tchong-Fou	LU	1
Zhongji	Chukyoku	Tchong-Tsi	CV	3
Zhongliao	Churyo	Tchong-Tsiao	BL	33
Zhonglushu	Churyoyu	Tchong-Liu-Iu	BL	29
Zhongshu	Chusu	Tchong-Tchroe	GV	7
Zhongting	Chutei	Tchong-Ting	CV	16
Zhongwan	Chukan	Tchong-Koann	CV	12
Zhongzhu	Chusho	Tchong-Tchou	TH	3
Zhongzhu	Chuchu	Tchong-Tchou	KI	15
Zhouliao	Churyo	Tcheou-Tsiao	LI	12
Zhourong	Shuei	Tcheou-Iong	SP	20
Zhubin	Chikuhin	Tso-Pinn	KI	9
Zigong	Shikyu	Tsre-Kong	CV	19
Zu Qiaoyin	Ashi no Korin	Tsiao-Inn	GB	44
Zusanli	Ashi no Sanri	Sann-Li	ST	36

P = Pinyin Chinese · J = Japanese
F = French · Ns = Numbered system

JAPANESE ALPHABETIZED

J	F	P	Ns	
Amon	Ia-Menn	Changqiang	GV	15
Ashi no Gori	Ou-Li	Zu Wuli	LV	10
Ashi no Kyoin	Tsiao-Inn	Zu-Qiaoyin	GB	44
Ashi no Rinkyu	Linn-Tsri	Zu-Linqi	GB	41
Ashi no Sanri	Sann-Li	Zusanli	ST	36
Ashi no Tsukoku	Trong-Kou	Tonggu	BL	66
Ashi no Yokan	Iang-Koann	Xiyangguan	GB	33
Atama no Kyoin	Tsiao-Inn	Qianoyin	GB	11
Atama no Rinkyu	Linn-Tsri	Linqi	GB	15
Bisho	Mei-Tchrong	Meichong	BL	3
Bokoyu	Prang-Koang-Iu	Pangguangshu	BL	28
Bokushin	Prou-Chenn	Pushen	BL	61
Chigoe	Ti-Ou-Roe	Diwuhui	GB	42
Chiki	Ti-Tsi	Diji	SP	8
Chikuhin	Tso-Pinn	Zhubin	KI	9
Chippen	Tche-Pienn	Zhibian	BL	49/54
Chiso	Tchreng-Tsri	Dicang	ST	4
Choe	Ting-Roe	Tinghui	GB	2
Chokin	Tchre-Tsinn	Zhejin	GB	23
Chokyo	Tchrang-Tsiang	Changqiang	GV	1
Chokyu	Ting-Kong	Tinggong	SI	19
Chuchu	Tchong-Tchou	Zhongzhu	KI	15
Chufu	Tchong-Fou	Zhongfu	LU	1
Chuho	Tchong-Fong	Zhongfeng	LV	4
Chukan	Tchong-koann	Zhongwan	CV	12
Chukyoku	Tchong-Tsi	Zhongji	CV	3

J = Japanese · F = French
P = Pinyin Chinese · Ns = Numbered system

J	F	P	Ns	
Churyo	Tchong-Tsiao	Zhongliao	BL	33
Churyo	Tcheou-Tsiao	Wuli	LI	12
Churyoyu	Tchong-Liu-Iu	Zhonglushu	BL	29
Chusho	Tchong-Tchou	Zhongzhu	TH	3
Chusho	Tchong-Tchrong	Zhongchong	CS	9
Chusu	Tchong-tchrou	Zhongshu	GV	7
Chutei	Tchong-Ting	Zhongting	CV	16
Chuto	Tchong-Tou	Zhongdu	LV	6
Chutoku	Sia-Tou	Zhongdu	GB	32
Daichoyu	Ta-Tchrang-Iu	Dachangshu	BL	25
Daigei	Se-Pae	Daying	ST	5
Daiho	Ta-Pao	Dabao	SP	21
Daijo	Ta-Tchrou	Dazhu	BL	11
Daikaku	Ta-Ro	Dahe	KI	12
Daiko	Ta-Tsiu	Daju	ST	27
Daio	Ta-Rong	Daheng	SP	15
Dairyo	Ta-Ling	Daling	CS	7
Daisho	Ta-Tchong	Dazhong	KI	4
Daito	Ta-Tou	Dadu	SP	2
Daiton	Ta-Toun	Dadun	LV	1
Daitsui	Pae-Lao	Dazhui	GV	14
Danchu	Trann-Tchong	Shangzhong	CV	17
Datan	Toe-Toann	Duduan	GV	27
Doshiryo	Trong-Tse-Tsiao	Tongziliao	GB	1
Eifu	I-Fong	Yifeng	TH	17
Ein	Roe-Inn	Huiyin	CV	1

J = Japanese · F = French
P = Pinyin Chinese · Ns = Numbered system

	J	F	P	Ns
	Ekimon	Ie-Menn	Yemen	TH 2
	Eneki	Iuann-Ie	Yuanye	GB 22
	Eso	Roe-Tsong	Huizong	TH 7
	Eyo	Roe-Iang	Huiyang	BL 35
	Fubun	Fou-Fenn	Fufen	BL 36/41
	Fuchi	Fong-Tchre	Fengchi	GB 20
	Fufu	Fong-Fou	Fengfu	GV 16
	Fugeki	Feou-Tsri	Fuxi	BL 52/38
	Fuhaku	Feou-pae	Fubai	GB 10
	Fukuai	Fou-Ngae	Fuai	SP 16
	Fukuryu	Fou-Leou	Fuliu	KI 7
	Fukuto	Fou-Trou	Futu	ST 32
	Fumon	Fong-Menn	Fengmen	BL 12
	Fusha	Fou-Che	Fushe	SP 13
	Fushi	Fong-Che	Fengshi	GB 31
	Futotsu	Fou-Trou	Heiliao	LI 18
	Fuyo	Pou-Jong	Burang	ST 19
	Fuyo	Fou-Iang	Fuyang	BL 59
	Gaikan	Oae-Koann	Waiguan	TH 5
	Gaikyu	Oae-Tsiou	Waiqiu	GB 36
	Gairyo	Oae-Ling	Wailing	ST 26
	Ganen	Rann-Ia	Waigiu	GB 4
	Geiko	Ing-Siang	Yingxiang	LI 20
	Gekan	Ti-Tsrang	Xiaguan	ST 7
Ekimon /	Gekan	Sia-Koann	Xiawan	CV 10
Gekimon	Gekimon	Tsri-Menn	Ximen	CS 4

J = Japanese · F = French
P = Pinyin Chinese · Ns = Numbered system

J	F	P	Ns	
Gekokyo	Sia-Lienn	Xiajuwu	ST	39
Geren	Sia-Lienn	Xialian	LI	8
Geryo	Sia-Tsiao	Xialiao	BL	34
Ginko	Inn-Tsiao	Yinjiao	GV	28
Gocho	Reou-Ting	Houding	GV	19
Gokei	Reou-Tsri	Houxi	SI	3
Gokoku	Ro-Kou	Hegu	LI	4
Gosho	Ou-Tchrou	Wuchu	BL	5
Gosu	Ou-Tchrou	Wushu	GB	27
Goyo	Ro-Iang	Heyang	BL	55
Gyokuchin	Iu-Tchenn	Yuzhen	BL	9
Gyokudo	Iu-Trang	Yutang	CV	18
Gyosai	Iu-Tsi	Yuji	LU	10
Haiyu	Fei-Iu	Feishu	BL	13
Hakkanyu	Pae-Roann-Iu	Baihuanshu	BL	30
Hakko	Pro-Rou	Pohu	BL	37/42
Hara no Tsukoku	Trong-Kou	Tonggu	KI	20
Heifu	Tchreng-Fong	Bingfeng	SI	12
Henreki	Pienn-Li	Pianli	LI	6
Hiju	Pi-Nao	Binao	LI	14
Hikan	Pi-Koann	Biguan	ST	31
Hiyo	Fei-Iang	Feiyang	BL	58
Hiyu	Pi-Iu	Pishu	BL	20
Hoko	Pao-Roang	Baohuang	BL	48/53
Honshin	Penn-Chenn	Benshen	GB	13
Horo	Pou-Lang	Bulang	KI	22

J = Japanese · F = French
P = Pinyin Chinese · Ns = Numbered system

J	F	P	Ns
Horyu	Fong-Long	Fenglong	ST 40
Hukketsu	Fou-Tsie	Fujie	SP 14
Hyakue	Pae-Roe	Baihui	GV 20
Ichu	Oe-Tchong	Weizhong	BL 54/40
Ido	Oe-Tao	Weidao	GB 28
Iki	I-Si	Yixi	BL 40/45
Impaku	Inn-Po	Yinbai	SP 1
Impo	Inn-Pao	Yinbao	LV 9
Ingeki	Inn-Tsri	Yinxi	HT 6
Inko	Inn-Tsiao	Yinjiao	CV 7
Inkoku	Inn-Kou	Yingu	KI 10
Inmon	Inn-Menn	Yinmen	BL 51/37
Inren	Inn-Lienn	Yinlian	LV 11
Inryosen	Inn-Ling-Tsiuann	Yinlingquan	SP 9
Inshi	Inn-Che	Yinshi	ST 33
Into	Inn-Tou	Yindu	KI 19
Isha	I-Che	Yishe	BL 44/49
Iso	Oe-Tsrang	Weicang	BL 45/50
Iyo	Oe-Iang	Weiyang	BL 53/39
Iyu	Oe-Iu	Weishu	BL 21
Jikan	El-Tsienn	Erjian	LI 2
Jimon	Se-Tchou-Kong	Ermen	TH 21
Jingei	Jenn-Ing	Renying	ST 9
Jinyu	Chenn-Iu	Sehshu	BL 23
Jiryo	Tsre-Tsiao	Ciliao	BL 32
Jitsugetsu	Je-Iue	Riyue	GB 24

J = Japanese · F = French
P = Pinyin Chinese · Ns = Numbered system

J	F	P	Ns	
Jokan	Chang-Koann	Shangwan	CV	13
Joko	Tiao-Kreou	Tiaokou	ST	38
Jokokyo	Chang-Lienn	Shangjuxu	ST	37
Joren	Chang-Lienn	Shanglian	LI	9
Joryo	Chang-Tsiao	Shangliao	BL	31
Josei	Chang-Sing	Shangxing	GV	23
Jue	Nao-Roe	Naohui	TH	13
Juyu	Nao-Iu	Naoshu	SI	10
Kagai	Roa-Kae	Huagai	CV	20
Kaikei	Tsie-Tsri	Jiexi	ST	41
Kakkan	Ko-Koann	Geguan	BL	41/46
Kakushujin	Kro-Tchou-Jenn	Shangguan	GB	3
Kakuson	Tsio-Soun	Jiaosun	TH	20
Kakuyu	Ko-Iu	Geshu	BL	17
Kancho	Roann-Tsiao	Huantiao	GB	30
Kangen	Koann-Iuann	Guanyuan	CV	4
Kangenyu	Koann-Iuann-Iu	Guanyuansho	BL	26
Kankoku	Sienn-Kou	Xiangu	ST	43
Kankotsu	Oann-Kou	Wangu	GB	12
Kanmon	Koann-Menn	Guanmen	ST	22
Kanshi	Tsienn-Che	Jiashi	CS	5
Kansyo	Koann-Tchrong	Guanchong	TH	1
Kanyu	Kann-Iu	Ganshu	BL	18
Karyo	Ro-Tsiao	Heiliao	LI	19
Katsunikumon	Roa-Jeou	Huaroumen	ST	24
Keikotsu	Tsing-Kou	Jinggu	BL	64

J = Japanese · F = French
P = Pinyin Chinese · Ns = Numbered system

J	F	P	Ns	
Keikyo	Tsing-Tsiu	Jingqu	LU	8
Keimon	Tsing-Menn	Jingmen	GB	25
Keimyaku	Tchre-Mo	Qimai	TH	18
Kekkai	Siue-Rae	Xuehai	SP	10
Kenchuyu	Tsienn-Tchong	Jianzhongshu	SI	15
Kengaiyu	Tsienn-Oae	Jianwaishu	SI	14
Kengu	Tsienn-Iu	Jianju	LI	15
Kenri	Tsienn-Li	Jianli	CV	11
Kenri	Siuann-Li	Xuanli	GB	6
Kenro	Siuann-Lou	Xuanlu	GB	5
Kenryo	Tsienn-Tsiao	Jianliao	TH	14
Kenryo	Tsiuann-Tsiao	Quanliao	SI	18
Kensei	Tienn-Tsing	Jianjing	GB	21
Kensho	Siuann-Tchong	Xuanzhong	GB	39
Kensu	Siuann-Tchrou	Xuanshu	GV	5
Kentei	Tsienn-Tchenn	Jianzhen	SI	9
Ketsubon	Tsiue-Prenn	Quepen	ST	12
Ketsuinyu	Tsiue-Inn-Iu	Jueyinshu	BL	14
Kikai	Tsri-Rae	Qihai	CV	6
Kikaiyu	Tsri-Rae-Iu	Qihaishu	BL	24
Kiketsu	Tsri-Tsiue	Qixue	KI	13
Kiko	Tsri-Rou	Qihu	ST	13
Kimon	Tsi-Menn	Jimen	SP	11
Kimon	Tsri-Menn	Qimen	LV	14
Kinmon	Tsinn-Menn	Jinmen	BL	63
Kinshuku	Tsinn-Chou	Jinsuo	GV	8

J = Japanese · F = French
P = Pinyin Chinese · Ns = Numbered system

J	F	P	Ns	
Kirai	Koe-Lae	Guilai	ST	29
Kisha	Tsri-Che	Qishe	ST	11
Kisho	Tsri-Tchrong	Qichong	ST	30
Kobo	Krou-Fang	Kufang	ST	14
Kokan	Sing-Tsienn	Xingjian	LV	2
Koketsu	Tsiu-Koann	Juque	CV	14
Koko	Kao-Roang	Luoque	BL	38/43
Kokotsu	Tsiu-Kou	Jugu	LI	16
Komei	Koang-Ming	Guangming	GB	37
Komon	Roang-Menn	Huangmen	BL	46/51
Konmon	Roun-Menn	Hunmen	BL	42/47
Konron	Kroun-Loun	Kunlun	BL	60
Koryo	Tsia-Tchre	Juliao	ST	3
Kosai	Krong-Tsoe	Kongzui	LU	6
Koshin	Tsiao-Sinn	Jiaoxin	KI	8
Koshi no Yokan	Iang-Koann	Yaoyangguan	GV	3
Koson	Kong-Soun	Gongsun	SP	4
Koyu	Roang-Iu	Huangshu	KI	16
Kyohaku	Sie-Po	Xiabai	LU	4
Kyokan	Tsiang-Tsienn	Qiangjian	GV	18
Kyokei	Sie-Tsri	Xiaxi	GB	43
Kyokkotsu	Tsiou-Kou	Qugu	CV	2
Kyokubin	Tsiou-Ping	Qubin	GB	7
Kyokuchi	Tsiou-Tchre	Quchi	LI	11
Kyokuen	Tsiou-Iuann	Xiaohai	SI	13
Kyokusa	Tsiou-Tchrae	Quchai	BL	4

J = Japanese · F = French
P = Pinyin Chinese · Ns = Numbered system

J	F	P	Ns	
Kyokusen	Tsi-Tsiuann	Jiquan	HT	1
Kyokusen	Tsiou-Tsiuann	Ququan	LV	8
Kyokutaku	Tsiou-Tsre	Quze	CS	3
Kyokyo	Siong-Siang	Xiongxiang	SP	19
Kyoryo	Tsiu-Tsiao	Juliao	GB	29
Kyosha	Tsiu-Tsiao	Jiache	ST	6
Kyubi	Tsiou-Oe	Jiuwei	CV	15
Kyukyo	Tsiou-Siu	Qiuxu	GB	40
Kyumyaku	Iang-Che	Jimai	LV	12
Meimon	Ming-Menn	Mingmen	GV	4
Mokuso	Mou-Tchroang	Muchuang	GB	16
Naikan	Nei-Koann	Neiguan	CS	6
Naitei	Nei-Ting	Neiting	ST	44
Nenkoku	Jenn-Kou	Rangu	KI	2
Noko	Nao-Rou	Nachu	GV	17
Noku	Nao-Krong	Naokong	GB	19
Nyuchu	Jou-Tchong	Ruzhong	ST	17
Nyukon	Jou-Kenn	Rugen	ST	18
Okotsu	Rong-Kou	Henggu	KI	11
Okuei	Ou-I	Wuyi	ST	15
Onryu	Oenn-Leou	Wenliu	LI	7
Rakkyaku	Lo-Tsri	Luoque	BL	8
Reida	Li-Toe	Lidui	ST	45
Reidai	Ling-Trae	Lingtai	GV	10
Reido	Ling-Tao	Lingdao	HT	4
Reiko	Li-Keou	Ligou	LV	5

J = Japanese · F = French
P = Pinyin Chinese · Ns = Numbered system

J	F	P	Ns	
Reikyo	Ling-Siu	Lingxu	KI	24
Rekketsu	Lie-Tsiue	Lieque	LU	7
Rensen	Lienn-Tsiuann	Lianquan	CV	23
Rokoku	Leou-Kou	Lougu	SP	7
Rokyu	Lao-Kong	Laogong	CS	8
Rosoku	Lou-Si	Luxi	TH	19
Ryokyu	Leang-Tsiou	Liangqiu	ST	34
Ryomon	Leang-Menn	Liangmen	ST	21
Sanchiku	Tsroann-Tchou	Zanzhu	BL	2
Saninko	Sann-Inn-Tsiao	Sanyinjiao	SP	6
Sankan	Sann-Tsienn	Sanjian	LI	3
Sanshoyu	Sann-Tsiao-Iu	Sanjiaoshu	BL	22
Sanyoraku	Sann-Iang-Lo	Sanyangluo	TH	8
Seimei	Tsing-Ming	Jingming	BL	1
Seirei	Tsring-Ling	Qingling	HT	2
Seireien	Tsring-Leng-Iuann	Qinglengyuan	TH	11
Sekichu	Tsi-Tchong	Jizhong	GV	6
Sekikan	Che-Koann	Shiguan	KI	18
Sekimon	Che-Menn	Shimen	CV	5
Senki	Siuann-Tsi	Xuanji	CV	21
Shakutaku	Tchre-Tsre	Chize	LU	5
Shichikuku	El-Menn	Sizhukong	TH	23
Shihaku	Sia-Koann	Sibai	ST	2
Shiin	Tche-Inn	Zhiyin	BL	67
Shiko	Tche-Keou	Zhigou	TH	6
Shikyu	Tsre-Kong	Zigong	CV	19

J = Japanese · F = French
P = Pinyin Chinese · Ns = Numbered system

J	F	P	Ns
Shiman	Se-Mann	Siman	KI 14
Shimpo	Chenn-Fong	Shenfeng	KI 23
Shinchu	Chenn-Tchou	Shenzhu	GV 12
Shindo	Chenn-Trang	Shentang	BL 39/44
Shindo	Chenn-Tao	Shendao	GV 11
Shine	Tchroang-Roe	Xinhui	GV 22
Shinketsu	Chenn-Koann	Shenque	CV 8
Shinmon	Chenn-Menn	Shenmen	HT 7
Shinmyaku	Chenn-Mo	Shenmai	BL 62
Shintei	Chenn-Ting	Shenting	GV 24
Shinyu	Sinn-Iu	Xinshu	BL 15
Shinzo	Chenn-Tsrang	Shencang	KI 25
Shisei	Tche-Tcheng	Zhizheng	SI 7
Shishitsu	Tche-Che	Zhishi	BL 47/52
Shitoku	Se-Tou	Sidu	TH 9
Shitsukan	Si-Koann	Xiguan	LV 7
Shiyo	Tche-Iang	Zhiyang	GV 9
Shochoyu	Siao-Tchrang-Iu	Xiaochangshu	BL 27
Shoei	Tcheng-Ing	Zhengying	GB 17
Shofu	Tchreng-Fou	Chengfu	BL 50/36
Shofu	Chao-Fou	Shaofu	HT 8
Shokai	Siao-Rae	Xiaohai	SI 8
Shokai	Tchao-Rae	Zhaohai	KI 6
Shokai	Chao-Rae	Shaohai	HT 3
Shokin	Tchreng-Tsinn	Chengjin	BL 56
Shoko	Tchreng-Koang	Chengguan	BL 6

J = Japanese · F = French
P = Pinyin Chinese · Ns = Numbered system

J	F	P	Ns	
Shokutoku	Che-Teou	Shidou	SP	17
Shokyoku	Chang-Tsiou	Shangqu	KI	17
Shokyu	Treou-Oe	Chengqi	ST	1
Shokyu	Chang-Tsiou	Shangqiu	SP	5
Shoman	Tchreng-Mann	Chengman	ST	20
Shomon	Tchrong-Menn	Chongmen	SP	12
Shomon	Tchang-Menn	Zhangmen	LV	13
Shorei	Tchreng-Ling	Chengling	GB	18
Shoreki	Siao-Lo	Xiaoluo	TH	12
Shosho	Tchreng-Tsiang	Chengjiang	CV	24
Shosho	Chao-Chang	Shaoshang	LU	11
Shosho	Chao-Tchrong	Shaochong	HT	9
Shotaku	Chao-Tsre	Shoatse	SI	1
Shoyo	Chang-Iang	Shangyang	LI	1
Shozan	Tchreng-Chann	Chengshan	BL	57
Shuei	Tcheou-Iong	Zhourong	SP	20
Sokkoku	Choae-Kou	Shuaigu	GB	8
Sokkotsu	Chou-Kou	Shugu	BL	65
Soryo	Sou-Tsiao	Suliao	GV	25
Suibun	Choe-Fenn	Shuifen	CV	9
Suido	Choe-Tao	Shuidao	ST	28
Suiko	Choe-Keou	Renzhong	GV	26
Suisen	Choe-Tsiuann	Shuiquan	KI	5
Suitotsu	Choe-Trou	Shuitu	ST	10
Syoyo	Tchrong-Iang	Chongyang	ST	42
Taien	Trae-Iuann	Taiyuan	LU	9

J = Japanese · F = French
P = Pinyin Chinese · Ns = Numbered system

J	F	P	Ns	
Taihaku	Trae-Po	Taibai	SP	3
Taiitsu	Trae-I	Taiyi	ST	23
Taikei	Trae-Tsri	Taixi	KI	3
Taimyaku	Tae-Mo	Daimai	GB	26
Taisho	Trae-Tchrong	Taichong	LV	3
Tanyu	Tann-Iu	Danshu	BL	19
Tempu	Tienn-Fou	Tianfu	LU	3
Tenchi	Tienn-Tchre	Tianchi	CS	1
Tenchu	Tienn-Tchou	Tianzhu	BL	10
Tenkei	Tienn-Tsri	Tianxi	SP	18
Te no Gori	Ou-Li	Wuli	LI	13
Te no Sanri	Sann-Li	Shousanli	LI	10
Tenryo	Tienn-Tsiao	Tianliao	TH	15
Tensei	Tienn-Tsing	Tianjing	TH	10
Tensen	Tienn-Tsiuann	Tianquan	CS	2
Tensho	Tienn-Tchrong	Tianchong	GB	9
Tenso	Tienn-Tsong	Tianzong	SI	11
Tenso	Tsienn-Tchroang	Tianchuang	SI	16
Tensu	Tienn-Tchrou	Tianshu	ST	25
Tentei	Tienn-Ting	Tianding	LI	17
Tentotsu	Tienn-Trou	Tiantu	CV	22
Tenyo	Tienn-Jong	Tianrong	SI	17
Tenyu	Tienn-Iou	Tianyou	TH	16
Todo	Trao-Tao	Taodao	GV	13
Tokubi	Tou-Pi	Dubi	ST	35

J = Japanese · F = French
P = Pinyin Chinese · Ns = Numbered system

J	F	P	Ns	
Tokuyu	Tou-Iu	Dushu	BL	16
Tsuri	Trong-Li	Tongli	HT	5
Tsuten	Trong-Tienn	Tongtian	BL	7
Unmon	Iunn-Menn	Yumen	LU	2
Wakuchu	Rouo-Tchong	Yuzhong	KI	26
Wankotsu	Oann-Kou	Wangu	SI	4
Waryo	Ro-Tsiao	Heliao	TH	22
Yochi	Iang-Tchre	Yangchi	TH	4
Yohaku	Iang-Pae	Yangbai	GB	14
Yoho	Iang-Fou	Yangfu	GB	38
Yokei	Iang-Tsri	Yangxi	LI	5
Yoko	Iang-Kang	Yanggang	BL	43/48
Yoko	Iang-Tsiao	Yangjiao	GB	35
Yokoku	Iang-Kou	Yanggu	SI	5
Yoro	Iang-Lao	Yanglao	SI	6
Yoryosen	Iang-Ling-Tsiuann	Yanglingquan	GB	34
Yoso	Ing-Tchroang	Yinchuang	ST	16
Yoyu	Iao-Iu	Yaoshu	GV	2
Yufu	Iu-Fou	Shufu	KI	27
Yumon	Iou-Menn	Youmen	KI	21
Yusen	Iong-Tsiuann	Yongquan	KI	1
Zencho	Tsienn-Ting	Qianding	GV	21
Zenkoku	Tsienn-Kou	Qiangu	SI	2
Zui	Ta-Ing	Touwei	ST	8

J = Japanese · F = French
P = Pinyin Chinese · Ns = Numbered system

FRENCH

ALPHABETIZED

F	P	J	Ns	
Cae-Tsiou	Waiqiu	Gaikyu	GB	36
Chang-Iang	Shangyang	Shoyo	LI	1
Chang-Koann	Shangwan	Jokan	CV	13
Chang-Lienn	Shanglian	Joren	LI	9
Chang-Lienn	Shangjuxu	Jokoyo	ST	37
Chang-Sing	Shangxing	Josei	GV	23
Chang-Tsiao	Shangliao	Joryo	BL	31
Chang-Tsiou	Shangqui	Shokyu	SP	5
Chang-Tsiou	Shangqu	Shokyoku	KI	17
Chao-Chang	Shaoshang	Shosho	LU	11
Chao-Fou	Shaochong	Shofu	HT	8
Chao-Rae	Shaohai	Shokai	HT	3
Chao-Tsre	Shaotse	Shaotaku	SI	1
Chao-Tsrong	Shaochong	Shosho	HT	9
Che-Koann	Shiguan	Sekikan	KI	18
Che-Menn	Shimen	Sekimon	CV	5
Che-Teou	Shidou	Shokutoku	SP	17
Chenn-Fong	Shenfeng	Shimpo	KI	23
Chenn-Iu	Shenshu	Jinyu	BL	23
Chenn-Koann	Shenque	Shinketsu	CV	8
Chenn-Menn	Shenmen	Shimon	HT	7
Chenn-Mo	Shenmai	Shinmyaku	BL	62
Chenn-Tao	Shendao	Shindo	GV	11
Chenn-Tchou	Shenzhu	Shinchu	GV	12
Chenn-Ting	Shenting	Shintai	GV	24
Chenn-Trang	Shentang	Shindo	BL	39/44

F = French • P = Pinyin Chinese
J = Japanese • Ns = Numbered system

F	P	J	Ns
Chenn-Tsrang	Shencang	Shinzo	KI 25
Choae-Kou	Shuaigu	Sokkoku	GB 8
Choe-Fenn	Shuifen	Suibun	CV 9
Choe-Keou	Suliao	Suiko	GV 26
Choe-Tao	Shuidao	Suido	ST 28
Choe-Trou	Shuitu	Suitotsu	ST 10
Choe-Tsiuann	Dazhong	Daisho	KI 5
Chou-Kou	Jinggu	Sokkotsu	BL 65
El-Menn	Sizhukong	Shichikuku	TH 23
El-Tsienn	Erjian	Jikan	LI 2
Fei-Iang	Feiyang	Hiyo	BL 58
Fei-Iu	Feishu	Haiyu	BL 13
Feou-Pae	Fubai	Fuhaku	GB 10
Feou-Tsri	Fuxi	Fugeki	BL 52/38
Fong-Che	Fengshi	Fushi	GB 31
Fong-Fou	Feng-fu	Fufu	GV 16
Fong-Long	Fenglong	Horyu	ST 40
Fong-Menn	Fengmen	Fumon	BL 12
Fong-Tchre	Fengchi	Fuchi	GB 20
Fou-Che	Fushe	Fusha	SP 13
Fou-Fenn	Fufen	Fubun	BL 36/41
Fou-Iang	Fuyang	Fuyo	BL 59
Fou-Leou	Fuliu	Fukuryu	KI 7
Fou-Ngae	Fuai	Fukuai	SP 16
Fou-Trou	Futu	Futotsu	LI 18
Fou-Trou	Futu	Fukuto	ST 32

F = French • P = Pinyin Chinese
J = Japanese • Ns = Numbered system

F	P	J	Ns	
Fou-Tsie	Fujie	Hukketsu	SP	14
I-Che	Yishe	Isha	BL	44/49
I-Fong	Yifeng	Eifu	TH	17
I-Si	Yixi	Iki	BL	40/45
Ia-Menn	Yamen	Amon	GV	15
Iang-Che	Jimai	Kyumyaku	LV	12
Iang-Fou	Yangfu	Yoho	GB	38
Iang-Kang	Yanggang	Yoko	BL	43/48
Iang-Koann	Yaoyangguan	Koshi no Yokan	GV	3
Iang-Kou	Yanggu	Yokoku	SI	5
Iang-Lao	Yanglao	Yoro	SI	6
Iang-Ling-Tsiuann	Yanglingquan	Yoryosen	GB	34
Iang-Pae	Benshen	Yohaku	GB	14
Iang-Tchre	Yangchi	Yochi	TH	4
Iang-Tsiao	Yangjiao	Yoko	GB	35
Iang-Tsri	Yangxi	Yokei	LI	5
Iao-Iu	Yaoshu	Yoyu	GV	2
Ie-Menn	Yemen	Ekimon	TH	2
Ing-Siang	Yingxiang	Geiko	LI	20
Ing-Tchroang	Yinchuang	Yoso	ST	16
Inn-Che	Yinshi	Inshi	ST	33
Inn-Kou	Yingu	Inkoku	KI	10
Inn-Lienn	Yinlian	Inren	LV	11
Inn-Ling-Tsiuann	Yinlingquan	Inryosen	SP	9
Inn-Menn	Yinmen	Inmon	BL	51/37
Inn-Pao	Yinbao	Impo	LV	9

F = French • P = Pinyin Chinese
J = Japanese • Ns = Numbered system

F	P	J	Ns	
Inn-Po	Yinbai	Impaku	SP	1
Inn-Tou	Yindu	Into	KI	19
Inn-Tsiao	Yinjiao	Inko	CV	7
Inn-Tsiao	Yinjiao	Ginko	GV	28
Inn-Tsri	Yinxi	Ingeki	HT	6
Iong-Tsiuann	Yongquan	Yusen	KI	1
Iou-Menn	Youmen	Yumon	KI	21
Iu-Fou	Shufu	Yufu	KI	27
Iu-Tchenn	Yuzhen	Gyokuchin	BL	9
Iu-Trang	Yutang	Gyokudo	CV	18
Iu-Tsi	Yuji	Gyosai	LU	10
Iuann-Ie	Yuanye	Eneki	GB	22
Iunn-Menn	Yunmen	Unmon	LU	2
Je-Iue	Riyue	Jitsugetsu	GB	24
Jenn-Ing	Renying	Jingei	ST	9
Jenn-Kou	Rangu	Nenkoku	KI	2
Jou-Kenn	Rugen	Nyukon	ST	18
Jou-Tchong	Ruzhong	Nyuchu	ST	17
Kann-Iu	Ganshu	Kanyu	BL	18
Kao-Roang	Gaohuang	Koko	BL	38/43
Ko-Iu	Geshu	Kakuyu	BL	17
Ko-Koann	Geguan	Kakkan	BL	41/46
Koang-Iuann-Iu	Guanyuanshu	Kangenyu	BL	26
Koang-Ming	Guangming	Komei	GB	37
Koann-Iuann	Guanyuan	Kangen	CV	4
Koann-Menn	Guanmen	Kanmon	ST	22

F = French • P = Pinyin Chinese
J = Japanese • Ns = Numbered system

F	P	J	Ns
Koann-Tchrong	Guanchong	Kansyo	TH 1
Koe-Lae	Guilai	Kirai	ST 29
Kong-Soun	Gongsun	Koson	SP 4
Kro-Tchou-Jenn	Shangguan	Kakushujin	GB 3
Krong-Tsoe	Kongzui	Kosai	LU 6
Krou-Fang	Kufang	Kobo	ST 14
Kroun-Loun	Kunlun	Konron	BL 60
Lao-Kong	Laogong	Rokyu	CS 8
Leang-Menn	Liangmen	Ryomon	ST 21
Leang-Tsiou	Liangqiu	Ryokyu	ST 34
Leou-Kou	Lougu	Rokoku	SP 7
Li-Keou	Ligou	Reiko	LV 5
Li-Toe	Lidui	Reida	ST 45
Lie-Tsiue	Lieque	Rekketsu	LU 7
Lienn-Tsiuann	Lianquan	Rensen	CV 23
Ling-Siu	Lingxu	Reikyo	KI 24
Ling-Tao	Lingdao	Reido	HT 4
Ling-Trae	Lingtai	Reidai	GV 10
Linn-Tsri	Linqi	Atama no Rinkyu	GB 15
Linn-Tsri	Zul-Linqi	Ashi no Rinkyu	GB 41
Lo-Tsri	Luoque	Rakkyaku	BL 8
Lou-Si	Luxi	Rosoku	TH 19
Mei-Tchrong	Meichong	Bisho	BL 3
Ming-Menn	Mingmen	Meimon	GV 4
Mou-Tchroang	Muchuang	Mokuso	GB 16
Nao-Iu	Naoshu	Juyu	SI 10
Nao-Krong	Naokong	Noku	GB 19
Nao-Roe	Naohui	Jue	TH 13

F = French • P = Pinyin Chinese
J = Japanese • Ns = Numbered system

F	P	J	Ns	
Nao-Rou	Naohu	Noko	GV	17
Nei-Koann	Neiguan	Naikan	CS	6
Nei-Ting	Neiting	Naitai	ST	44
Oae-Koann	Waiguan	Gaikan	TH	5
Oae-Ling	Wailing	Gairyo	ST	26
Oae-Tsiou	Waiqiu	Gaikyu	GB	36
Oann-Kou	Wangu	Wankotsu	SI	4
Oann-Kou	Wangu	Kankotsu	GB	12
Oe-Iang	Weiyang	Iyo	BL	53/39
Oe-Iu	Weishu	Iyu	BL	21
Oe-Tao	Juliao	Ido	GB	28
Oe-Tchong	Weizhong	Ichu	BL	54/40
Oe-Tsrang	Weicang	Iso	BL	45/50
Oenn-Leou	Wenliu	Onryu	LI	7
Ou-I	Wuyi	Okuei	ST	15
Ou-Li	Wuli	Te no Gori	LI	13
Ou-Li	Wuli	Ashi no Gori	LV	10
Ou-Tchrou	Wuchu	Gosho	BL	5
Ou-Tchrou	Wushu	Gosu	GB	27
Pae-Lao	Dazhui	Daitsui	GV	14
Pae-Roann-Iu	Baihuanshu	Hakkanyu	BL	30
Pae-Roe	Baihui	Hyakue	GV	20
Pao-Roang	Baohuang	Hoko	BL	48/53
Penn-Chenn	Benshen	Honshin	GB	13
Pi-Iu	Pishu	Hiyu	BL	20
Pi-Koann	Biguan	Hikan	ST	31
Pi-Nao	Binao	Hiju	LI	14
Pienn-Li	Pianli	Henreki	LI	6

F = French • P = Pinyin Chinese
J = Japanese • Ns = Numbered system

F	P	J	Ns	
Pou-Jong	Burang	Fuyo	ST	19
Pou-Lang	Bulang	Horo	KI	22
Prang-Koang-Iu	Pangguangshu	Bokoyu	BL	28
Pro-Rou	Pohu	Hakko	BL	37/42
Prou-Chenn	Pushen	Bokushin	BL	61
Rann-Ia	Hanyan	Ganen	GB	4
Reou-Ting	Houding	Gocho	GV	19
Reou-Tsri	Houxi	Gokei	SI	3
Ro-Iang	Heyang	Goyo	BL	55
Ro-Kou	Hegu	Gokoku	LI	4
Ro-Tsiao	Nose-Heliao	Karyo	LI	19
Ro-Tsiao	Heliao	Waryo	TH	22
Roa-Jeou	Huaroumen	Katsunikumon	ST	24
Roa-Kae	Huagai	Kagai	CV	20
Roang-Iu	Huangshu	Koyu	KI	16
Roang-Menn	Huangmen	Komon	BL	46/51
Roann-Tsiao	Huantiao	Kancho	GB	30
Roe-Iang	Gaohuang	Eyo	BL	35
Roe-Inn	Huyin	Ein	CV	1
Roe-Tsong	Qubin	Eso	TH	7
Rong-Kou	Henggu	Okotsu	KI	11
Roun-Menn	Hunmen	Konmon	BL	42/47
Rouo-Tchong	Yuzhong	Watuchu	KI	26
Sann-Iang-Lo	Sanyangluo	Sanyoraku	TH	8
Sann-Inn-Tsiao	Sanyinjiao	Saninko	SP	6
Sann-Li	Shousanli	Te no Sanri	LI	10

F = French • P = Pinyin Chinese
J = Japanese • Ns = Numbered system

F	P	J	Ns	
Sann-Li	Zusanli	Ashi no Sanri	ST	36
Sann-Tsiao-Iu	Sanjiaoshu	Sanshoyu	BL	22
Sann-Tsienn	Sanjian	Sankan	LI	3
Se-Mann	Siman	Shiman	KI	14
Se-Pae	Daying	Daigei	ST	5
Se-Tchou-Kong	Ermen	Jimon	TH	21
Se-Tou	Sidu	Shitoku	TH	9
Si-Koann	Qubin	Shitsukan	LV	7
Sia-Koann	Erjian	Shihaku	ST	2
Sia-Koann	Xiawan	Gekan	CV	10
Sia-Lienn	Xialian	Geren	LI	8
Sia-Lienn	Xiajuxu	Gekokyo	ST	39
Siao-Lo	Xiaoluo	Shoreki	TH	12
Siao-Rae	Xiaohai	Shokai	SI	8
Siao-Tchrang-Iu	Xiaochangshu	Shochoyu	BL	27
Sia-Tou	Zhongdu	Chutoku	GB	32
Sia-Tsiao	Xialiao	Geryo	BL	34
Sie-Po	Xiabai	Kyohaku	LU	4
Sie-Tsri	Xiaxi	Kyokei	GB	43
Sienn-Kou	Xiangu	Kankoku	ST	43
Sing-Tsienn	Xingjian	Kokan	LV	2
Sinn-Iu	Xinshu	Shinyu	BL	15
Siong-Siang	Xiongsiang	Kyokyo	SP	19
Siuann-Li	Xuanli	Kenri	GB	6
Siuann-Lou	Xuanlu	Kenro	GB	5
Siuann-Tchong	Xuanzhong	Kensho	GB	39

F = French • P = Pinyin Chinese
J = Japanese • Ns = Numbered system

F	P	J	Ns
Siuann-Tchrou	Xuanshu	Kensu	GV 5
Siuann-Tsi	Xuanji	Senki	CV 21
Siue-Rae	Xuehai	Kekai	SP 10
Sou-Tsiao	Suliao	Soryo	GV 25
Ta-Ing	Touwei	Zui	ST 8
Ta-Ling	Daling	Dairyo	CS 7
Ta-Pao	Dabao	Daiho	SP 21
Ta-Ro	Dahe	Daikaku	KI 12
Ta-Rong	Daheng	Daio	SP 15
Ta-Tchong	Dazhong	Daisho	KI 4
Ta-Tchrang-Iu	Dachangshu	Daichoyu	BL 25
Ta-Tchrou	Dazhu	Daijo	BL 11
Ta-Tou	Dadu	Daito	SP 2
Ta-Toun	Dadun	Daiton	LV 1
Ta-Tsiu	Daju	Daiko	ST 27
Tae-Mo	Daimai	Taimyaku	GB 26
Tann-Iu	Danshu	Tanyu	BL 19
Tchang-Menn	Zhangmen	Shomon	LV 13
Tchao-Rae	Zhaohai	Shokai	KI 6
Tche-Che	Zhishi	Shishitsu	BL 47/52
Tche-Iang	Zhiyang	Shiyo	GV 9
Tche-Inn	Zhiyin	Shiin	BL 67
Tche-Keou	Zhigou	Shiko	TH 6
Tche-Pienn	Zhibian	Chippen	BL 49/ 54
Tche-Tcheng	Zhizheng	Shisei	SI 7
Tcheng-Ing	Zhengying	Shoei	GB 17
Tcheou-Iong	Zhourong	Shuei	SP 20

Siuann-Tchrou / Tcheou- Iong

F = French • P = Pinyin Chinese
J = Japanese • Ns = Numbered system

F	P	J	Ns	
Tcheou-Tsiao	Zhouliao	Churyo	LI	12
Tchong-Fong	Zhongfeng	Chuho	LV	4
Tchong-Fou	Zhongfu	Chufu	LU	1
Tchong-Koann	Zhongwan	Chukan	CV	12
Tchong-Liu-Iu	Zhonglushu	Churyoyu	BL	29
Tchong-Tchou	Zhongzhu	Chuchu	KI	15
Tchong-Tchou	Zhongzhu	Chusho	TH	3
Tchong-Tchrong	Zhongchong	Chusho	CS	9
Tchong-Tchrou	Zhongshu	Chusu	GV	7
Tchong-Ting	Zhongting	Chutei	CV	16
Tchong-Tou	Zhongdu	Chuto	LV	6
Tchong-Tsi	Zhongji	Chukyoku	CV	3
Tchong-Tsiao	Zhongliao	Churyo	BL	33
Tchrang-Tsiang	Changqiang	Chokyo	GV	1
Tchre-Mo	Qimai	Keimyaku	TH	18
Tchre-Tsinn	Zhejin	Chokin	GB	23
Tchre-Tsre	Chize	Shakutaku	LU	5
Tchreng-Chann	Chengshan	Shozan	BL	57
Tchreng-Fong	Dahe	Heifu	SI	12
Tchreng-Fou	Chengfu	Shofu	BL	50/36
Tchreng-Koang	Chengguang	Shoko	BL	6
Tchreng-Ling	Chengling	Shorei	GB	18
Tchreng-Mann	Chengman	Shoman	ST	20
Tchreng-Tsiang	Chengchiang	Shosho	CV	24
Tchreng-Tsinn	Chengjin	Shokin	BL	56
Tchreng-Tsri	Dicang	Chiso	ST	4

F = French • P = Pinyin Chinese
J = Japanese • Ns = Numbered system

F	P	J	Ns
Tchroang-Iang	Chongyang	Syoyo	ST 42
Tchroang-Roe	Xinhui	Shine	GV 22
Tchrong-Menn	Chongmen	Shomon	SP 12
Ti-Ou-Roe	Diwuhui	Chigoe	GB 42
Ti-Tsi	Diji	Chiki	SP 8
Ti-Tsrang	Xiaguan	Gekan	ST 7
Tiao-Kreou	Tiaokou	Joko	ST 38
Tienn-Fou	Tianfu	Tempu	LU 3
Tienn-Iou	Tianyou	Tenyu	TH 16
Tienn-Jong	Tianrong	Tenyo	SI 17
Tienn-Tchou	Tianzhu	Tenchu	BL 10
Tienn-Tchre	Tianchi	Tenchi	CS 1
Tienn-Tchroang	Tianchuang	Tenso	SI 16
Tienn-Tchrong	Tianchong	Tensho	GB 9
Tienn-Tchrou	Tianshu	Tensu	ST 25
Tienn-Ting	Tianding	Tentei	LI 17
Tienn-Trou	Tiantu	Tentotsu	CV 22
Tienn-Tsiao	Tianliao	Tenryo	TH 15
Tienn-Tsing	Tianjing	Tensei	TH 10
Tienn-Tsing	Jianjing	Kensei	GB 21
Tienn-Tsiuann	Tianquan	Tensen	CS 2
Tienn-Tsong	Tianzong	Tenso	SI 11
Tienn-Tsri	Tianxi	Tenkei	SP 18
Ting-Kong	Tinggong	Chokyu	SI 19
Ting-Roe	Tinghui	Choe	GB 2
Toe-Toann	Duduan	Datan	GV 27

F = French • P = Pinyin Chinese
J = Japanese • Ns = Numbered system

F	P	J	Ns	
Tou-Iu	Dushu	Tokuyu	BL	16
Tou-Pi	Dubi	Tokubi	ST	35
Trae-I	Taiyi	Taiitsu	ST	23
Trae-Iuann	Taiyuan	Taien	LU	9
Trae-Po	Taibai	Taihaku	SP	3
Trae-Tchrong	Taichong	Taisho	LV	3
Trae-Tsri	Taixi	Taikei	KI	3
Trann-Tchong	Shaozhong	Danchu	CV	17
Trao-Tao	Taodao	Todo	GV	13
Treou-Oe	Chenggai	Shokyu	ST	1
Trong-Kou	Zhiyin	Ashi no Tsukoku	BL	66
Trong-Kou	Tonggu	Hara no Tsukoku	KI	20
Trong-Li	Tongli	Tsuri	HT	5
Trong-Tienn	Tongtian	Tsuten	BL	7
Trong-Tse-Tsiao	Tongziliao	Doshiryo	GB	1
Tsi-Menn	Jimen	Kimon	SP	11
Tsi-Tchong	Jizhong	Sekichu	GV	6
Tsi-Tsiuann	Jiquan	Kyokusen	HT	1
Tsia-Tchre	Juliao	Kor yo	ST	3
Tsiang-Tsienn	Qiangjian	Kyokan	GV	18
Tsiao-Inn	Qiaoyin	Ashi no Kyoin	GB	44
Tsiao-Inn	Qiaoyin	Atama no Kyoin	GB	11
Tsiao-Sinn	Shiguan	Koshin	KI	8
Tsie-Tsri	Kaikei	Kaikei	ST	41
Tsienn-Che	Jianshi	Kanshi	CS	5
Tsienn-Iu	Jianju	Kengu	LI	15

F = French • P = Pinyin Chinese
J = Japanese • Ns = Numbered system

F	P	J	Ns
Tsienn-Kou	Qianqu	Zenkoku	SI 2
Tsienn-Li	Jianli	Kenri	CV 11
Tsienn-Oae	Jianwaishu	Kengaiyu	SI 14
Tsienn-Tchenn	Tinggong	Kentai	SI 9
Tsienn-Tchong	Jianzhongshu	Kenchuyu	SI 15
Tsienn-Tchroang	Tianchuang	Tenso	SI 16
Tsienn-Ting	Qianding	Zencho	GV 21
Tsienn-Tsiao	Jianliao	Kenryo	TH 14
Tsienn-Tsiao	Tianliao	Tenryo	TH 15
Tsing-Kou	Jinggu	Keikotsu	BL 64
Tsing-Menn	Jingmen	Keimon	GB 25
Tsing-Ming	Jingmen	Seimei	BL 1
Tsing-Tsiu	Jingqu	Keikyo	LU 8
Tsinn-Chou	Jingsuo	Kinshuku	GV 8
Tsinn-Menn	Tonggu	Kinmon	BL 63
Tsio-Soun	Jiaosun	Kakuson	TH 20
Tsiou-Iuann	Quyuan	Kyokuen	SI 13
Tsiou-Kou	Ququ	Kyokkotsu	CV 2
Tsiou-Oe	Jiuwei	Kyubi	CV 15
Tsiou-Ping	Qubin	Kyokubin	GB 7
Tsiou-Siu	Qiuxu	Kyukyo	GB 40
Tsiou-Tchrae	Quchai	Kyokusa	BL 4
Tsiou-Tchre	Quchi	Kyokuchi	LI 11

F = French • P = Pinyin Chinese
J = Japanese • Ns = Numbered system

F	P	J	Ns	
Tsiou-Tsiuann	Ququan	Kyokusen	LV	8
Tsiou-Tsre	Zhongji	Kyokutaku	CS	3
Tsiu-Koann	Juque	Koketsu	CV	14
Tsiu-Kou	Jugu	Koktsu	LI	16
Tsiu-Tsiao	Jiache	Kyosha	ST	6
Tsiu-Tsiao	Juliao	Kyoryo	GB	29
Tsiuann-Tsiao	Quanliao	Kanryo	SI	18
Tsiue-Inn-Iu	Jueyinshu	Ketsuinyu	BL	14
Tsiue-Prenn	Quepen	Ketsubon	ST	12
Tso-Pinn	Zhubin	Chikuhin	KI	9
Tsre-Kong	Shikyu	Shikyu	CV	19
Tsre-Tsiao	Ciliao	Jiryo	BL	32
Tsri-Che	Qishe	Kisha	ST	11
Tsri-Menn	Qimen	Kimon	LV	14
Tsri-Menn	Ximen	Gekimon	CS	4
Tsri-Rae	Neiguan	Kikai	CV	6
Tsri-Rae-Iu	Qihaishu	Kikaiyu	BL	24
Tsri-Rou	Qihu	Kiko	ST	13
Tsri-Tchrong	Qichong	Kisho	ST	30
Tsri-Tsiue	Qixue	Kiketsu	KI	13
Tsring-Ling	Qingling	Seirei	HT	2
Tsring-Ling-Iuann	Qinglengyuan	Seireisen	TH	11
Tsroann-Tchou	Jingming	Sanchiku	BL	2

F = French • P = Pinyin Chinese
J = Japanese • Ns = Numbered system

WADE-GILES

CHINESE

ALPHABETIZED

Name	Meridian	Point
Changchiang	GV	1
Changmen	LV	13
Chaohai	KI	6
Chechin	GB	23
Chengchi	ST	1
Chengchiang	CV	24
Chengchin	BL	56
Chengfu	BL	50/36
Chengkuang	BL	6
Chengling	GB	18
Chengman	ST	20
Chengshan	BL	57
Chengying	GB	17
Chiache	ST	6
Chiangchien	GV	18
Chiaohsin	KI	8
Chichuan	HT	1
Chichung	GV	6
Chichung	ST	30
Chiehhsi	ST	41
Chienchen	SI	9
Chienching	GB	21
Chienchungshu	SI	15
Chienku	SI	2
Chienli	CV	11
Chienliao	TH	14
Chienshih	CS	5
Chienting	GV	21
Chienwaishu	SI	14
Chienyu	LI	15
Chihai	CV	6
Chihaishu	BL	24
Chihcheng	SI	7
Chihkou	TH	6
Chihmo	TH	18
Chihpien	BL	49/54
Chihshih	BL	47/52
Chihsueh	KI	13
Chihtse	LU	5
Chihu	ST	13
Chihyang	GV	9
Chihyin	BL	67
Chingchu	LU	8
Chingku	BL	64
Chinglengyuan	TH	11
Chimen	LV	14
Chimen	SP	11
Chimo	LV	12
Chingling	HT	2
Chingmen	GB	25
Chingming	BL	1
Chinmen	BL	63
Chinso	GV	8
Chishe	ST	11
Chiuhsu	GB	40
Chiuwei	CV	15
Chongmen	SP	12
Chouliao	LI	12
Chouyung	SP	20
Chuanliao	SI	18
Chucha	BL	4
Chuchih	LI	11
Chuchuan	LV	8
Chuchueh	CV	14
Chuehpen	ST	12
Chuehsun	TH	20
Chuehyinshu	BL	14
Chuku	CV	2
Chuku	LI	16
Chuliao	GB	29
Chuliao	ST	3
Chungchi	CV	3
Chungchung	CS	9
Chungchu	TH	3
Chungchu	KI	15
Chungfeng	LV	4
Chungfu	LU	1
Chungliao	BL	33
Chunglushu	BL	29
Chungshu	GV	7
Chungting	CV	16
Chungtu	GB	32
Chungtu	LV	6
Chungwan	CV	12
Chungyang	ST	42
Chupin	GB	7
Chupin	KI	9
Chutse	CS	3
Chuyuan	SI	13
Erhchien	LI	2
Erhmen	TH	21
Feishu	BL	13
Feiyang	BL	58

Fengchih	GB	20
Fengfu	GV	16
Fenglung	ST	40
Fengmen	BL	12
Fengshih	GB	31
Fuai	SP	16
Fuchieh	SP	14
Fufen	BL	36/41
Fuhsi	BL	52/38
Fuliu	KI	7
Fupai	GB	10
Fushe	SP	13
Futu	ST	32
Futu	LI	18
Fu Tungku	KI	20
Fuyang	BL	59
Hanyen	GB	4
Hengku	KI	11
Heyang	BL	55
Holiao	TH	22
Holiao	LI	19
Hoku	LI	4
Houhsi	SI	3
Houting	GV	19
Hsiachuhsu	ST	39
Hsiahsi	GB	43
Hsiakuan	ST	7
Hsialiao	BL	34
Hsialien	LI	8
Hsiaochangshu	BL	27
Hsiaohai	SI	8
Hsiaolo	TH	12
Hsiapai	LU	4
Hsiawan	CV	10
Hsienku	ST	43
Hsikuan	LV	7
Hsimen	CS	4
Hsingchien	LV	2
Hsinhui	GV	22
Hsinshu	BL	15
Hsiunghsiang	SP	19
Hsuanchi	CV	21
Hsuanchung	GB	39
Hsuanli	GB	6
Hsuanlu	GB	5
Hsuanshu	GV	5
Hsuehhai	SP	10
Huajoumen	ST	24
Huakai	CV	20
Huangmen	BL	46/51
Huangshu	KI	16
Huantiao	GB	30
Huitsung	TH	7
Huiyang	BL	35
Huiyin	CV	1
Hunmen	BL	42/47
Janku	KI	2
Jenchung	GV	26
Jenying	ST	9
Jihyueh	GB	24
Juchung	ST	17
Juken	ST	18
Kanshu	BL	18
Kaohuang	BL	38/43
Kekuan	BL	41/46
Keshu	BL	17
Kuanchong	TH	1
Kuangming	GB	37
Kuanmen	ST	22
Kuanyuan	CV	4
Kuanyuanshu	BL	26
Kueilai	ST	29
Kufang	ST	14
Kungsun	SP	4
Kungtsui	LU	6
Kunlun	BL	60
Laokung	CS	8
Liangchiu	ST	34
Liangmen	ST	21
Liehchueh	LU	7
Lienchuan	CV	23
Likou	LV	5
Linghsu	K	24
Lingtai	GV	10
Lingtao	HT	4
Litui	ST	45
Lochueh	BL	8
Louku	SP	7
Luhsi	TH	19
Meichung	BL	3
Mingmen	GV	4
Muchuang	GB	16
Naohu	GV	17

Name	Meridian	Point
Naohui	TH	13
Naokung	GB	19
Naoshu	SI	10
Neikuan	CS	6
Neiting	ST	44
Paihuanshu	BL	30
Paihui	GV	20
Pangkuangshu	BL	28
Paohuang	BL	48/53
Penshen	GB	13
Pienli	LI	6
Pikuan	ST	31
Pinao	LI	14
Pingfeng	SI	12
Pishu	BL	20
Pohu	BL	37/42
Pulang	KI	22
Pushen	BL	61
Puyung	ST	19
Sanchiaoshu	BL	22
Sanchien	LI	3
Sanyanglo	TH	8
Sanyinchiao	SP	6
Shanchung	CV	17
Shangchiu	SP	5
Shangchu	KI	17
Shangchuhsu	ST	37
Shanghsing	GV	23
Shangkuan	GB	3
Shangliao	BL	31
Shanglien	LI	9
Shangyang	LI	1
Shanwan	CV	13
Shaochung	HT	9
Shaofu	HT	8
Shaohai	HT	3
Shaoshang	LU	11
Shaotse	SI	1
Shenchu	GV	12
Shenchueh	CV	8
Shenfeng	KI	23
Shenmen	HT	7
Shenmo	BL	62
Shenshu	BL	23
Shentang	BL	39/4
Shentao	GV	11
Shenting	GV	24
Shentsang	K	25
Shihkuan	K	18
Shihmen	CV	5
Shihtou	SP	17
Shousanli	LI	10
Shouwuli	LI	13
Shuaiku	GB	8
Shufu	KI	27
Shuichuan	KI	5
Shuifen	CV	9
Shuitao	ST	28
Shuitu	ST	10
Shuku	BL	65
Ssuchukung	TH	23
Suliao	GV	25
Szuman	KI	14
Szupai	ST	2
Szutu	TH	9
Tachangshu	BL	25
Tachu	BL	11
Tachu	ST	27
Tachui	GV	14
Tachung	KI	4
Taheng	SP	15
Taichung	LV	3
Taihsi	KI	3
Taimo	GB	26
Taipai	SP	3
Taiyi	ST	23
Taiyuan	LU	9
Taheh	KI	12
Taling	CS	7
Tanshu	BL	19
Taotao	GV	13
Tapao	SP	21
Tatu	SP	2
Tatun	LV	1
Taying	ST	5
Tiaokou	ST	38
Tichi	SP	8
Tienchih	CS	1
Tienching	TH	10
Tienchu	BL	10

Name	Meridian	Point
Tienchuan	CS	2
Tienchuang	SI	16
Tienchung	GB	9
Tienfu	LU	3
Tienhsi	SP	18
Tienjung	SI	17
Tienliao	TH	15
Tienshu	ST	25
Tienting	LI	17
Tientsung	SI	11
Tientu	CV	22
Tienyu	TH	16
Tinghui	GB	2
Tingkung	SI	19
Titsang	ST	4
Tiwuhui	GB	42
Tou chiaoyin	GB	11
Tou Linchi	GB	15
Touwei	ST	8
Tsanchu	BL	2
Tsu Chiaoyin	GB	44
Tsu Linchi	GB	41
Tsusanli	ST	36
Tsu tungku	BL	66
Tsuwuli	LV	10
Tsu Yangkuan	GB	33
Tuituan	GV	27
Tungli	HT	5
Tungtien	BL	7
Tungtzuliao	GB	1
Tupi	ST	35
Tushu	BL	16
Tzukung	CV	19
Tzuliao	BL	32
Waichiu	GB	36
Waikuan	TH	5
Wailing	ST	26
Wanku	GB	12
Wanku	SI	4
Weichung	BL	54/40
Weishu	BL	21
Weitao	GB	28
Weitsang	BL	45/50
Weiyang	BL	53/39
Wenliu	LI	7
Wuchu	BL	5
Wushu	GB	27
Wuyi	ST	15
Yamen	GV	15
Yangchiao	GB	35
Yangchih	TH	4
Yangfu	GB	38
Yangkang	BL	43/48
Yangku	SI	5
Yanglao	SI	6
Yanglingchuan	GB	34
Yangpai	GB	14
Yangsi	LI	5
Yaoshu	GV	2
Yao Yangkuan	GV	3
Yemen	TH	2
Yifeng	TH	17
Yihsi	BL	40/45
Yinchiao	GV	28
Yinchiao	CV	7
Yingchuang	ST	16
Yinghsiang	LI	20
Yinhsi	HT	6
Yinku	KI	10
Yinlien	LV	11
Yinlingchuan	SP	9
Yinmen	BL	51/37
Yinpai	SP	1
Yinpao	LV	9
Yintu	KI	19
Yinshih	ST	33
Yishe	BL	44/49
Yuanyeh	GB	22
Yuchen	BL	9
Yuchi	LU	10
Yuchung	KI	26
Yumen	KI	21
Yungchuan	KI	1
Yunmen	LU	2
Yutang	CV	18

ENGLISH TRANSLATION OF CHINESE CHARACTERS

N	W	O	L	O & B
Heart Meridian				
I.1	Extreme source	1st draining pt. of spring	polar fountain	Summit's Spring
I.2	Blue-green	blue spirits	pure soul	Youthful spirit
I.3	Little sea	entrance to the ocean	little sea	Lesser Sea
I.4	Spirit pathway	heart spirit pathway	way of soul	Spirit's Path
I.5	Penetrating inside	junction point	accessible village	Reaching the Measure
I.6	Yin mound	impact point	Yin fissure	Yin Xi
I.7	Spirit gate	gate of God	spiritual door	Spirit's Door
I.8	Lesser palace	entrance of the capital	little residence	Lesser Residence
I.9	Little rushing in	little impact	small thoroughfare	Lesser Pouring
Small Intestine Meridian				
II.1	Little marsh	beginning of the stream	little marsh	Lesser Marsh
II.2	Forward valley	front valley	frontal valley	Forward Valley
II.3	Back ravine	back stream	creek at rear	Back Creek
II.4	Wrist bone	wrist bone	wrist bone	Wrist Bone
II.5	Yang valley	yang valley	yang valley	Valley of Yang
II.6	Supporting the old	revitalizing the old	for retirement	Nourish the Old
II.7	Upright branch	upstraight pivot	center of branches	Branch of Uprightness
II.8	Small sea	entrance of the energy ocean	small sea	Small Sea
II.9	Upright shoulder	pivot of the shoulder	lower shoulder	Shoulder Chastity

N = Numbered System • W = Worsley • O = Ohashi
L = Lu • O & B = O'Connor & Bensky

N	W	O	L	O & B
II.10	Shoulder blade	shoulder point	medial upper arm transport	Scapula's Hollow
II.11	Heavenly ancestor	center in the heaven	heavenly clans	Heaven's Ancestor
II.12	Grasping the wind	facing the wind	natural wind	Holding Wind
II.13	Crooked wall	fence on the corner	bending wall	Crooked Wall
II.14	Outside of the shoulder correspondence	outside of shoulder yu	lateral transport of shoulder	Shoulder's Outer Hollow
II.15	Middle of the shoulder correspondence	middle of shoulder yu	medial transport of shoulder	Mid-Shoulder Hollow
II.16	Heavenly window	heaven's window	heavenly window	Heaven's Window
II.17	Heavenly appearance	heaven's container	heavenly capacity	Heaven's Contents
II.18	Cheek bone	cheek bone	zygomatic foramen	Cheek Seam
II.19	Listening palace	palace of hearing	palace of hearing	Palace of Hearing

Bladder Meridian

N	W	O	L	O & B
III.1	Eyes bright	bright light	clear vision	Eyes Bright
III.2	Collect bamboo	walking stick	bamboos collection	Gathered bamboo
III.3	Eyebrows rushing	above the eyebrow	eyebrow thoroughfare	Eyebrow's Pouring
III.4	Crooked servant	on the margin	winding discrepancy	Discrepancy
III.5	Five places	five places	five places	Five Places
III.6	Receive light	receiving light	inherited light	Support Light
III.7	Penetrate heaven	pass thru to the heaven	pass to heaven	Reaching Heaven
III.8	Lou end	connecting point	backward link	Decline

N = Numbered System • W= Worsley • O = Ohashi
L = Lu • O & B = O'Connor & Bensky

N	W	O	L	O & B
III.9	Jade pillow	jade pillow hitting pt.	jade occiput	Jade Pillow
III.10	Heavenly pillar	atlas pillar	heavenly pole	Heaven's Pillar
III.11	Great shuttle	important energy shuttle pt.	large shuttle	Big Shuttle
III.12	Wind gate	gate of wind	door to wind	Wind's Door
III.13	Lungs correspondence	lung yu	lung transport	Lung's Hollow
III.14	Absolute yin correspondence	heart constrictor yu	decreasing yin transport	Absolute Yin Hollow
III.15	Heart correspondence	heart yu	heart transport	Heart's Hollow
III.16	Governor correspondence	governor vessel yu	axis transport	Governing Hollow
III.17	Diaphragm correspondence	diaphragm yu	diaphragm transport	Diaphragm's Hollow
III.18	Liver correspondence	liver yu	liver transport	Liver's Hollow
III.19	Gall correspondence	gall bladder yu	gall transport	Gall Bladder's Hollow
III.20	Spleen correspondence	spleen yu	spleen transport	Spleen's Hollow
III.21	Stomach correspondence	stomach yu	stomach transport	Stomach's Hollow
III.22	Three heater correspondence	triple heater yu	triple burning transport	Triple Burner's Hollow
III.23	Kidneys correspondence	kidney yu	kidneys transport	Kidney's Hollow
III.24	Sea of Ch'i correspondence	ocean of ki yu	sea of energy transport	Sea of Qi Hollow
III.25	Large intestine correspondence	large intestine yu	large intestine transport	Large Intestine's Hollow
III.26	First gate correspondence	first gate yu	first gate transport	Hollow at the Hinge of the Source
III.27	Small intestine correspondence	small intestine yu	small intestine transport	Small Intestine's Hollow
III.28	Bladder correspondence	bladder yu	bladder transport	Bladder's Hollow
III.29	Middle of backbone correspondence	middle of back point	middle spinal erector transport	Mid-Spine Hollow

N = Numbered System • W = Worsley • O = Ohashi
L = Lu • O & B = O'Connor & Bensky

N	W	O	L	O & B
III.30	White ring correspondence	white ring point	white ring transport	White Circle's Hollow
III.31	Upper sacral bone	upper sacral hole	upper foramen	Eight Seams
III.32	Second sacral bone	second sacral hole	second foramen	Eight Seams
III.33	Middle sacral bone	middle sacral hole	middle foramen	Eight Seams
III.34	Lower sacral bone	lower sacral hole	lower foramen	Eight Seams
III.35	Meeting of Yang	meeting of Yang	meeting of Yang	Meeting of Yang
III.36	Near division	bifurcating point	subordinate part	Appended Part
III.37	Soul door	soul door	house of physical strength	Soul's Household
III.38	Rich for the vital correspondence	incurable disease point	heart & diaphragm	Vital's Hollow
III.39	Spirit hall	palace of God	spiritual hall	Spirit's Hall
III.40	Cry of pain	disaster & pain pt.	alas	Surprise
III.41	Diaphragm border	diaphragm point	diaphragm gate	Diaphram's Hinge
III.42	Spiritual soul gate	gate of the guts	door to soul	Soul's Door
III.43	Yang net	Yang net	Yang net	Yang's Parameter
III.44	Thought dwelling	mansion of will	sentiment residence	Will's Residence
III.45	Stomach granary	stomach granary	stomach storage	Stomach's Storehouse
III.46	Heart diaphragm gate	gate of vitality	diaphragm door	Vital's Door
III.47	Ambition room	chamber of ambition	will room	Will's Dwelling
III.48	Womb & heart diaphragm	womb vital point	womb diaphragm	Placenta and Vitals
III.49	Orderly frontier	folding edge	orderly edge	Order's Edge
III.50	Receive & support	receiving & support	heritary support	Receive Support
III.51	Prosperous gate	gate of Yin dynasty	middle door	Door of Abundance
III.52	Floating reserve	floating impact	floating fissure	Floating Xi

N = Numbered System • W = Worsley • O = Ohashi
L = Lu • O & B = O'Connor & Bensky

N	W	O	L	O & B
III.53	Equilibrium Yang	commanding Yang	impotent Yang	Commission the Yang
III.54	Equilibrium middle	center of commanding	bending center	Commission the Middle
III.55	Uniting Yang	uniting Yang	meeting of Yang	Confluence of Yang
III.56	Supporting muscles	supporting muscle	herited tendons	Support Sinews
III.57	Supporting mountain	supporting mountain	heritary mountain	Support the mountain
III.58	Fly & scatter	flying Yang	high position	Soaring
III.59	Foot bone Yang	Yang in the ankle	tarsal Yang	Tarsal Yang
III.60	Kun Lun mountains	Kun Lun mountains	mount Kun Lun	Kunlun Mountains
III.61	Servants aide	servant's aide	falling trio	Serve and Consult
III.62	Extended meridian	extending meridian	extended pulse	Extending Vessel
III.63	Golden gate	golden gate	golden door	Golden Door
III.64	Capital bone	main bone	tuberosity of 5th MT bone	Capital Bone
III.65	Bone binder	bone binder	head of 5th MT bone	Restraining Bone
III.66	Penetrating the valley	penetrating the valley	open-end valley	Connecting Valley of the Foot
III.67	Extremity of Yin	extremity of Yin	Yin in the extreme	End of Yin

Kidney Meridian

N	W	O	L	O & B
IV.1	Bubbling spring	gushing spring	bubbling fountain	Gushing Spring
IV.2	Blazing valley	blazing valley	burning valley	Burning Valley
IV.3	Greater mt. stream	great brook	great river	Great Creek
IV.4	Water spring	big bell	great bell	Big Goblet
IV.5	Great bell	water spring	water fountain	Spring

N = Numbered System • W = Worsley • O = Ohashi
L = Lu • O & B = O'Connor & Bensky

N	W	O	L	O & B
IV.6	Illuminated sea	deflecting ocean	dazzling sea	Shining Sea
IV.7	Returning current	returning current	returned stream	Returning Column
IV.8	Exchange pledges	exchanging correspondence	exchange of confidence	Communicate Belief
IV.9	Building guest	building the dunes	building of guest chamber	House Guest
IV.10	Yin valley	Yin valley	Yin valley	Yin's Valley
IV.11	Transverse bone	transverse pubis bone	transverse bone	Horizontal Bone
IV.12	Great brightness	great brightness	great glory	Great Clarity
IV.13	Door of infants	ki hole	energy point	Qi's Orifice
IV.14	Four full	four satisfaction	four in full	Four Full
IV.15	Middle flowing our	middle injection	middle transfusion	Middle Flow
IV.16	Intestinal correspondence	vital point	diaphragm transport	Vital's Hollow
IV.17	Merchant crooked	merchant on the corner	commercial winding	Trade Bend
IV.18	Stone border	stone gate	stone gate	Stone Hinge
IV.19	Yin capital	Yin capital	Yin capital	Yin's Metropolis
IV.20	Through the valley	through the valley	abdominal open-end valley	Connecting Valley on the Abdomen
IV.21	Dark gate	gate of the ghost	pylorus	Secluded Door (Pylorus)
IV.22	Walking on the verandah	walking corridor	walking veranda	Stepping Corridor
IV.23	Spirit seal	spirit-God seal	spiritual appointment	Spirit's Seal
IV.24	Spirit burial ground	spiritual burial ground	soul fair	Spirit's Ruins
IV.25	Spirit storehouse	spirit-God storehouse	spiritual hideout	Spirit's Storage
IV.26	Amidst elegance	amidst elegance	elegant center	Amid Elegance
IV.27	Store house	Yu mansion	transport house	Hollow Residence

N = Numbered System • W = Worsley • O = Ohashi
L = Lu • O & B = O'Connor & Bensky

N	W	O	L	O & B
Circulation-Sex Meridian				
V.1	Heavenly pond	heaven's pond	heavenly pond	Heaven's Pool
V.2	Heavenly spring	heaven's spring	heavenly fountain	Heaven's Spring
V.3	Crooked marsh	marsh on the corner	bending marsh	Crooked Marsh
V.4	Gate of Ch'i reserve	gate of impact	adjacent door	Gate of the Crevice
V.5	The intermediary	intermediary	messenger	Intermediary
V.6	Inner frontier gate	inner gate	inner gate	Inner Gate
V.7	Great mound	big mound	great mound	Big Tomb
V.8	Palace of weariness	palace of anxiety	palace of labor	Labor's Palace
V.9	Rushing into the middle	middle rushing	pulse in the middle finger	Middle Pouring
Three-Heater Meridian				
VI.1	Rushing the frontier gate	exit of the rushing energy	gate thoroughfare	Gate's Pouring
VI.2	Fluid secretion gate	gate of liquid	door to liquid	Fluid's Door
VI.3	Middle islet	middle islet	middle islet	Middle Island
VI.4	Yang pond	Yang pond	Yang pond	Pool of Yang
VI.5	Outer frontier gate	outer gate	outer gate	Outer Gate
VI.6	Branch ditch	divided ditch	branching ditch	Branch Ditch
VI.7	Assembly of ancestors	meeting of ancestor	meeting of the clans	Meeting of the Clan
VI.8	Three Yang junction	3 Yang meridian junction	link of three Yangs	Three Yang Connection
VI.9	Fourth gutter	four gutter	four gutters	Four Ditch

N = Numbered System • W = Worsley • O = Ohashi
L = Lu • O & B = O'Connor & Bensky

N	W	O	L	O & B
VI.10	Heavenly well	well in the heaven	heavenly well	Heaven's Well
VI.11	Pure cold abyss	pure cold abyss	clear & cold gulf	Cooling Gulf
VI.12	Relax and joy	tranquillity & joy	disappearing river	Melting Luo River
VI.13	Shoulder meeting	meeting pt. in the shoulder	meeting of upper arm	Shoulder's Meeting
VI.14	Shoulder bone	shoulder bone	under shoulder	Shoulder Seam
VI.15	Heavenly bone	heaven's bone	heavenly foramen	Heaven's Seam
VI.16	Heavenly window	window of the heaven	heavenly window	Heaven's Window
VI.17	Wind screen	wind screen	fan wind	Shielding Wind
VI.18	Feeding meridians	feeding meridian	abnormal pulse	Feeding the Vessels
VI.19	Skull breathing	skull breathing	cranial breath	Skull's Rest
VI.20	Small angle of ear	small angle of ear	angular grandchild	Angle of Regeneration
VI.21	Ear gate	gate of ear	door to ear	Ear's Door
VI.22	Harmony bone	harmony bone	peaceful foramen	Harmony Seam
VI.23	Silk bamboo hollow	silk bamboo hollow	tiny bamboo hole	Silken Bamboo Hollow

Gall Bladder Meridian

N	W	O	L	O & B
VII.1	Orbit bone	eye bone	pupil foramen	Pupil Seam
VII.2	Hearing assembly	hearing assembly	hearing center	Confluence of Hearing
VII.3	Upper pass	guest & host	upper gate	Upper Hinge
VII.4	Loathsome jaws	jaw detested	disagreeable chin	Jaw's Dislike
VII.5	Suspended skull	suspended skull	hanging brain	Suspended Skull
VII.6	Suspended regulator	suspended balance	suspended tx	Suspended Millimeter

N = Numbered System • W= Worsley • O = Ohashi
L = Lu • O & B = O'Connor & Bensky

N	W	O	L	O & B
VII.7	Crooked hair on the temples	hair on margin of temples	curled hair on the temples	Crook of the Temple
VII.8	Flowing valley	leading valley	in the valley	Leading to the Valley
VII.9	Heaven rushing	heaven rushing	heavenly thoroughfare	Heaven's Pouring
VII.10	Floating white	floating white	floating white	Floating White
VII.11	Head hole Yin	head extreme Yin	cavity of Yin	Yin Cavity on the Head
VII.12	Final bone	final bone	finished bone	Finished Bone
VII.13	Root spirit	root spirit	original spirit	Original Spirit
VII.14	Yang white	Yang white	sun white	Yang white
VII.15	Head above tears	good for tears	crying head	Near Tears on the Head
VII.16	Eye window	eye window	eye window	Vision's Window
VII.17	True Yin	honest business	regular camp	Upright Encampment
VII.18	Receiving spirit	receiving spirits	inherited soul	Support the Spirit
VII.19	Brain hollow	brain hollow	cranial cavity	Brain Cavity
VII.20	Wind pond	wind pond	wind pond	Pool of Wind
VII.21	Shoulder well	well in the shoulder	shoulder well	Shoulder well
VII.22	Arm-pit abyss	arm pit abyss	gulf fluids	Gull's Fluids
VII.23	Neglected muscles	neglected muscle	side tendons	Flank's Sinews
VII.24	Sun and moon	sun and moon	sun and moon	Sun Moon
VII.25	Capital gate	gate of the capital	capital door	Capital's door
VII.26	Girdle vessel	waistband extra meridian	belt pulse	Girdle Vessel
VII.27	Five pivots	five pivots	five pivots	Five Pivots
VII.28	Binding path	binding path	maintenance road	Maintain the Way
VII.29	Dwelling in the bone	dwelling in the bone	residing foramen	Stationary Seam
VII.30	Jumping circle	jumping pivot	jumping round	Encircling Leap

N = Numbered System • W= Worsley • O = Ohashi
L = Lu • O & B = O'Connor & Bensky

N	W	O	L	O & B
VII.31	Wind market	market of wind	city of wind	Wind's Market
VII.32	Middle ditch	middle ditch	central river	Middle Ditch
VII.33	Knee Yang border	Yang gate	Yang gate of knee	Knee's Yang Hinge
VII.34	Yang mound spring	Yang mound spring	mound fountain of Yang	Yang Tomb Spring
VII.35	Yang crossing	Yang crossing	connection of Yang	Yang's Intersection
VII.36	Outer mound	outer mound	lateral mound	Outer Mound
VII.37	Bright & clear	bright light	shiny & bright	Bright Light
VII.38	Yang support	Yang support	Yang assistant	Yang's Help
VII.39	Hanging cup	hanging bell	hanging cup	Suspended Time
VII.40	Wilderness mound	wilderness light	mound village	Mound of Ruins
VII.41	Foot above tears	good for tears	crying foot	Near Tears on the Foot
VII.42	Earth five meetings	earth five meetings	five meetings of earth	Ground's Fifth Meeting
VII.43	Valiant stream	narrow stream	rescue creek	Gallantry's Stream
VII.44	Foot hole Yin	Yin foot hole	Yin foramen of foot	Yin Cavity on the Foot

Liver Meridian

N	W	O	L	O & B
VIII.1	Great esteem	big origin point	great sincerity	Great Honesty
VIII.2	Walk between	in between	walking space	Walk Between
VIII.3	Supreme rushing	big rushing	great thoroughfare	Great Pouring
VIII.4	Middle seal	middle seal	middle mound	Middle Seal
VIII.5	Insect ditch	insect ditch	insect ditch	Worm Eater's Groove
VIII.6	Middle capital	middle capital	central capital	Middle Metropolis

---

N = Numbered System • W = Worsley • O = Ohashi
L = Lu • O & B = O'Connor & Bensky

N	W	O	L	O & B
VIII.7	Knee border	knee gate	knee gate	Knee's Hinge
VIII.8	Crooked spring	spring on the corner	bending fountain	Crooked Spring
VIII.9	Yin wrapping	Yin wrapping	Yin parcel	Yin's Wrapping
VIII.10	Five miles	five miles	five miles	Five Measures on the Foot
VIII.11	Yin angle	Yin screen	purity of Yin	Yin's Modesty
VIII.12	Hasty pulse	fast pulse	rapid pulse	Urgent Pulse
VIII.13	Chapter gate	distinguished gate	statutory door	System's Door
VIII.14	Gate of hope	gate of hope	centennial door	Expectation's Door

Lung Meridian

N	W	O	L	O & B
IX.1	Middle palace	energy coming in	central hall	Central Residence
IX.2	Cloud gate	cloud gate	cloud door	Cloud's Gate
IX.3	Heavenly palace	capital of heaven	heavenly door	Heaven's Residence
IX.4	Valiant White	surrounding white	charming white	Gallantry
IX.5	Outside marsh	indentation in the stream	pulse in the arm	Cubit Marsh
IX.6	Greatest hole	most energy gathering spot	foramen extreme	Opening Maximum
IX.7	Narrow defile	extreme shortcoming	eminent vacancy or electricity	Broken Sequence
IX.8	Meridian gutter	gutter in the meridian	flowing gutter	Across the Ditch
IX.9	Very great abyss	great gutter	great gulf	Great Abyss
IX.10	Fish region	edge of fish torso	fish line	Fish Border
IX.11	Little Merchant	end of lung element	scanty business	Lesser Merchant

N = Numbered System • W = Worsley • O = Ohashi
L = Lu • O & B = O'Connor & Bensky

N	W	O	L	O & B
Large Intestine Meridian				
X.1	Merchant Yang	Yang meridian starting pt. of metal element	commercial sunlight	Trade Yang
X.2	Second interval	2nd joint point	second space	Between Two
X.3	Third interval	3rd joint point	third space	Between Three
X.4	Joining of the valleys	valley meeting point	meeting of the valleys	Adjoining Valleys
X.5	Yang stream	sudden fall in Yang meridian	Yang river	Yang Creek
X.6	Side passage	distorted passage	inclined road	Partial Order
X.7	Warm current	warm well	warm current	Warm Slide
X.8	Lower side	lower corner	lower purity	Lower Integrity
X.9	Upper angle	upper corner	upper purity	Upper Integrity
X.10	Arm three miles	arm three miles	hand three miles	Arm's Three Measures
X.11	Crooked pond	pond on the corner	crooked pond	Crooked Pool
X.12	Elbow bone	elbow bone	under elbow	Elbow's Seam
X.13	Five miles	five miles	hand five miles	Five Measures on the Arm
X.14	Outer bone of the arm	all arm point	medial upper arm	Arm and Scapula
X.15	Shoulder bone	shoulder corner	shoulder joint	Shoulder Bone
X.16	Great bone	big bone	big bone	Great Bone
X.17	Heavenly vessel	controlling headquarter	heavenly strength	Heaven's Vessel
X.18	Support & rush out	supporting impact	supporting process	Support the Prominence
X.19	Grain bone	grain bone	growing foramen	Grain Seam
X.20	Welcome fragrance	welcome smell	greeting scent	Welcome Fragrance

N = Numbered System • W = Worsley • O = Ohashi
L = Lu • O & B = O'Connor & Bensky

N	W	O	L	O & B
Stomach Meridian				
XI.1	Receive tears	receiving tears	next to tears	Contain Tears
XI.2	Four whites	indentation point	four whites	Four Whites
XI.3	Great cheekbone	point on big bone	great foramen	Great Seam
XI.4	Earth granary	supply of the product of the earth	earth storage	Earth Granary
XI.5	Great welcome	big welcome	great welcome	Big Welcome
XI.6	Mandible wheel	pivot of the jaw	angle of the jaw	Jaw Vehicle
XI.7	Lower passage	lower gate	lower gate	Lower Hinge
XI.8	Head tied	corner of the head	head maintenance	Head Support
XI.9	People welcome	human welcome point	greetings of man	Man's Welcome
XI.10	Water rushing out	gate at the water	water process	Water Prominence
XI.11	Ch'i cottage	boarding house of rotten ki	energy residence	Qi's Residence
XI.12	Broken bowl	broken plate	supraclavicular fossa	Empty Basin
XI.13	Ch'i door	door of ki energy	energy house	Qi's Household
XI.14	Storehouse	storehouse	storage room	Storehouse
XI.15	Room screen	screen of the house	house fan	Room Screen
XI.16	Breast window	window of the chest	mamillary window	Breast's Window
XI.17	Center of the breasts	center of the nipple	breast center	Middle of Breast
XI.18	Root of the breasts	root of the breast	root of nipple	Breast's Root
XI.19	Not at ease	entrance pt of ST.	no capacity	Uncontainable
XI.20	Receiving fullness	receiving satisfaction	inherited fullness	Support Fullness
XI.21	Bridge gate	beam of the stomach	beam door	Door of the Beam

N = Numbered System • W = Worsley • O = Ohashi
L = Lu • O & B = O'Connor & Bensky

N	W	O	L	O & B
XI.22	Border gate	entrance gate	gate door	Gate
XI.23	Great oneness	oneness	divine star	Great Yi
XI.24	Lubrication food gate	gate of bone & muscle	sliding door of flesh	Door of Slippery Flesh
XI.25	Heavenly pivot	center of borderline	the north star	Heaven's Axis
XI.26	Outside mound	outside edge	lateral mound	Outer Tomb
XI.27	Great might	great point	tremendous greatness	The Great
XI.28	Water path	water road	waterway	Waterway
XI.29	The return	coming back point	coming back	Return
XI.30	Rushing order	ki energy impact pt.	thoroughfare of energy	Pouring Qi
XI.31	Thigh border	growing jt. point	gate of great trochanter	Hip's Hinge
XI.32	Prostrate hare	rabbit is lying down	hidden rabbit	Hidden Rabbit
XI.33	Yin market	chronic disease marketplace	Yin city	Yin's Market
XI.34	Beam mound	on the hill	timber mound	Ridge Mound
XI.35	Calf nose	calf nose	lateral knee eye	Eyes of Knees
XI.36	Leg three miles	leg three miles	foot three miles	Three Measures on the Knee
XI.37	Upper great void	upper great void	upper great emptiness	Upper void
XI.38	Branch opening	exit of the line	narrow mouth	Line's Opening
XI.39	Lower great void	lower great void	lower great emptiness	Lower Void
XI.40	Abundant splendor	abundant bulge	abundant protuberance	Abundance and Prosperity
XI.41	Released stream	ending stream point	melted creek	Release Stream
XI.42	Rushing Yang	impact of Yang	thoroughfare of Yang	Pouring Void
XI.43	Sinking valley	indented valley	depressed valley	Sinking Valley
XI.44	Inner courtyard	inner garden	inner yard	Inner Court
XI.45	Hard bargain	stimulating stomach meridian	bitter exchange	Strict Exchange

N = Numbered System • W = Worsley • O = Ohashi
L = Lu • O & B = O'Connor & Bensky

N	W	O	L	O & B

Spleen Meridian

N	W	O	L	O & B
XII.1	Retired white	inside white point	hidden white	Hidden White
XII.2	Great capital	big capital	great capital	Big Metropolis
XII.3	Supreme white	big indentation point	great white of Venus	Most White
XII.4	Princess grandson	grandchild	public grandchild	Grandfather's Grandson
XII.5	Merchant mound	metal point	commercial mounds	Mound of Commerce
XII.6	Three Yin crossing	meeting of three Yin leg meridians	meeting of three Yins	Three Yin Junction
XII.7	Leaky valley	leaking valley	leaking valley	Seeping Valley
XII.8	Earth motivator	earth source point	earth machine	Earth's Mechanism
XII.9	Yin mound spring	Yin mountain pond	mound fountain of Yin	Yin Tomb Spring
XII.10	Sea of blood	ocean of blood	sea of blood	Sea of Blood
XII.11	Basket gate	gate in the basket	transverse bone	
XII.12	Rushing gate	gate of impact	door to thoroughfare	Pouring Door
XII.13	Storehouse cottage	storehouse cottage	official residence	Dwelling
XII.14	Abdomen knot	abdomen knot	abdominal fruits	Abdomen's Knot
XII.15	Great horizontal	big horizontal	great pubis	Big Horizontal
XII.16	Abdomen sorrow	abdomen sorrow	abdominal misery	Abdomen's Sorrow
XII.17	Food drain	food drain	food drain	Food's Cavity
XII.18	Heavenly stream	entrance of heaven's energy	heavenly creek	Heaven's Stream
XII.19	Chest region	home of the chest village	chest town	Chest Home
XII.20	Encircling glory	surrounding prosperity	all-round honor	Encircling Glory
XII.21	Great enveloping	big enveloping	large parcel	Big Wrapping

N = Numbered System • W = Worsley • O = Ohashi
L = Lu • O & B = O'Connor & Bensky

N	W	O	L	O & B
Conception Vessel				
XIII.1	Meeting of Yin	meeting Yin	meeting of Yin	Perineum
XIII.2	Crooked bone	on the bone	bent bone	Crooked bone
XIII.3	Utmost middle	utmost center	middle point	Middle Summit
XIII.4	Border origin	gate of origin	first gate	Hinge of the Source
XIII.5	Stone gate	gate of stone	stone door	Stone Door
XIII.6	Sea of Ch'i	ocean of ki energy	sea of energy	Sea of Qi
XIII.7	Yin crossing	Yin crossing	connection of Yin	Yin's Junction
XIII.8	Spirit deficiency	spirit-God shrine	palace of Gods	Middle of the Navel
XIII.9	Water division	water division	juice or moisture	Water Part
XIII.10	Lower duct	lower duct	lower duct	Lower Cavity
XIII.11	Established mile	established mile	construction of village	Establish Measure
XIII.12	Middle duct	middle duct	middle duct	Middle Cavity
XIII.13	Upper duct	upper duct	upper duct	Upper Cavity
XIII.14	Great deficiency	great balcony	great imperial city	Great Palace
XIII.15	Dove tail	dove tail	pigeon tail	Wills Pigeon's Tail
XIII.16	Middle hall	middle courtyard	middle yard	Middle Hall
XIII.17	Within the breast	middle of the platform	middle pt. between nipples	Penetrating Odor
XIII.18	Jade court	jade court	jade hall	Jade court
XIII.19	Purple palace	purple palace	purple palace	Purple Palace
XIII.20	Flower covering	splendor covering	nine stars	Lustrous Cover
XIII.21	Pearl jade	pearl jade	fourth big dipper	North Star

N = Numbered System • W = Worsley • O = Ohashi
L = Lu • O & B = O'Connor & Bensky

N	W	O	L	O & B
XIII.22	Heaven rushing out	heaven impact	heavenly process	Heaven's Prominence
XIII.23	Angle spring	screen of spring	pure fountain	Modesty's Spring
XIII.24	Receiving fluid	receiving the drop of the water	mentolabial groove	Contain Fluid

Governor Vessel

N	W	O	L	O & B
XIV.1	Long strength	long & strong	long & strong	Long Strength
XIV.2	Loins correspondence	hip point	lumbar transport	Lower Back's Hollow
XIV.3	Loins Yang border	Yang gate	gate of Yang	Lumbar Yang's Hinge
XIV.4	Gate of life	gate of life	life door	Life's Door
XIV.5	Suspended pivot	hanging center	suspended center	Suspended Axis
XIV.6	Middle of the spine	center of vertebra	spinal center	Middle of Spine
XIV.7	Middle pivot	center of center	center	Middle Axis
XIV.8	Contracted muscle	contraction of tendon	tendon shrinking	Sinew's Shrinking
XIV.9	Extreme Yang	extreme Yang	Yang in the extreme	Reaching Yang
XIV.10	Supernatural tower	podium of speech	soul tower	Spirit's Platform

N = Numbered System • W = Worsley • O = Ohashi
L = Lu • O & B = O'Connor & Bensky

N	W	O	L	O & B
XIV.11	Spirit path	road of the God	spiritual way	Spirit's Path
XIV.12	Body pillar	pillar of the body	body pole	Body's Pillar
XIV.13	Kiln path	path of ceramic	clay door	Way of Happiness
XIV.14	Great hammer	big vertebra	great vertebra	Big Vertebra
XIV.15	Gate of dumbness	gate of dumb	door to mutism	Door of Muteness
XIV.16	Wind palace	capital of wind	palace of wind	Wind's Dwelling
XIV.17	Brain door	brain shelter	brain residence	Brain's Household
XIV.18	Strength divider	strength in between	strong envoy	Between Strength
XIV.19	Posterior summit	posterior summit	posterior vortex	Behind Top
XIV.20	One hundred meetings	hundred meetings	gatherings of hundred	Hundred meetings
XIV.21	Anterior summit	anterior summit	frontal vortex	Before Top
XIV.22	Skull meetings	skull meeting	meeting of fontanel	Fontanel's Meeting
XIV.23	Upper star	upper star	upper star	Upper Star
XIV.24	Spirit hall	spirit-God courtyard	spiritual yard	Spirit's Hall
XIV.25	Plain bone	plain bone	tip of nose	Plain Seam
XIV.26	Middle of the man	center of human	philtrum	Philtrum
XIV.27	Correct exchange	extreme end	tip of philtrum	Exchange Terminus
XIV.28	Mouth crossing	mouth closing	meeting of gums	Gum's Junction

N = Numbered System • W = Worsley • O = Ohashi
L = Lu • O & B = O'Connor & Bensky

Titles of the Twelve Primary Meridians

Eight Extra Meridians

Internal and Connecting Meridians

Unit of Measurement

Seven Radicals

Shu Points

Bibliography

I. Heart

P Cor Meridian (C)
W-G Shou Shao Yin Hsin Ching (H)
J Te No Shōinshinkei
K Su-so-um Sim Gyeong
F Méridien de Coeur (C)
G Herz-Meridian (H)
R Меридиан сердца
V Tam-Kinh
L Cardinalis Cardialis Yin Minoris Manus (cC)
E English alt: Lesser Yin, End of Yin, Yin Minimum, Arm lesser Yin, Heart Channel

II. Small Intestine

P Intestinum Tenue Meridian (IT)
W-G Shou t'tai-yang-hsiao-ch'ang-ching (Si)
J Te no Taiyōshōchōkei
K Su-Tae-Yang So Jang Gyeong
F Méridien de I'Intestin Grêle (G)
G Dunndarm-Meridian (DU)
R Меридиан тонкой кишки
V Tieu Truong Kinh
L Cardinalis Intestini Tenuis Yang Maioris Manus (cIT)
E Greater Yang, Big Yang, Large Yang, Arm Greater Yang, Small Intestine Channel

III. Bladder

P Vesica Urinaria Meridian (VU)
W-G Tsu Tai Yang Pang Kuang Ching (B)
J Ashi no Taiyobōkōkei
K Jog-Tae-Yang Bang-Gwang-Gyeong
F Méridien de la Vessie (V)
G Blasen Meridian (B)
R Меридиан мочевого пузыря
V Bang-Quang Kinh
L Cardinalis Vesicalis Yang Maioris Pedis (cV)
E Greater Yang, Big Yang, Large Yang, Leg Greater Yang, Bladder Channel

IV. Kidney

P Ren Meridian (R)
W-G Tsu Shao Yin Shen Ching (K)
J Ashi no Shōinjinkei
K Jog-So Eum-Sin-Gyeong
F Méridien des Reins (R)
G Nieren-Meridian (N)
R Меридиан почек
V Than Kinh
L Cardinalis Renalis Yin Minoris Pedis (cR)
E Lesser Yin, End of Yin, Yin Minimum, Leg Lesser Yin, Kidney Channel

---

P = Pinyin Chinese · W-G = Wade-Giles Chinese · J = Japanese
K = Korean · F = French · G = German · R = Russian
V = Vietnamese · L = Latin · E = English

V. Circulation-sex

P Pericardium Meridian (PC)
W-G Shou Chueh Yin Hsin Pao Ching (CX)
J Te no Ketsuinshimpōkei
K Su-Gweol-Eum-Sim-Po-Gyeong
F Méridien du Maître-du-coeur (MC)
G Meridian, Meister des Herzens (MH)
R Меридиан перикарда
V Tam Bao Lac
L Cardinalis Pericardialis Yin Flectentis Manus (cPC)
E Pericardium, Heart Constrictor, Heart Protector, Absolute Yin, Small Yin, Little Yin, Yin Equilibrium, Arm Absolute Yin, Pericardium Channel

VI. Three Heater

P Sanjiao Meridian (SJ)
W-G Shou Shoa Yang San Chiao Ching (T)
J Te no Syōyōsanshōkei
K Su-so-Yang-Sam Sho-Gyeong
F Méridien des Trois Rechauffeurs (TR)
G Meridian, Dreifacher Erwarmer (3E)
R Меридиан трех частей туловища
V Tam-Tieu Kinh
L Cardinalis Tricalorii Yang Minoris Manus (cT)
E Triple Heater, Triple Warmer, Tri Heater, Lesser Yang, Small Yang, Arm Lesser Yang, Triple Burner Channel

VII. Gall Bladder

P Vesica Fellea Meridian (VF)
W-G Tsu Shao Yang Tan Ching (G)
J Ashi no Shōyōtankei
K Jag-So-Yang-Dam-Gyeong
F Méridien de la Vésicule Biliaire (VB)
G Gallenblasen Meridian (G)
R Меридиан желчного пузыря
V Kinh Dom
L Cardinalis Fellea Yang Minoris Pedis (cF)
E Lesser Yang, Small Yang, Leg Lesser Yang, Gall Bladder Channel

VIII. Liver

P Hepar Meridian (H)
W-G Tsu Chueh Yin Kan Ching (LIV)
J Ashi no Ketsuinkankei
K Jog-Gweol-Eum-Gan-Gyeong
F Méridien du Foie (F)
G Leber-Meridian (LE)
R Меридиан печени
V Can Kinh
L Cardinalis Hepatica Yin Flectentis Pedis (cH)
E Absolute Yin, Small Yin, Little Yin, Yin Equilibrium, Leg Absolute Yin, Liver Channel

P = Pinyin Chinese · W-G = Wade-Giles Chinese · J = Japanese
K = Korean · F = French · G = German · R = Russian
V = Vietnamese · L = Latin · E = English

IX. Lung

P Pulmo Meridian (P)
W-G Shou Tai Yin Fei Ching (L)
J Te no Taiinhaikei
K Su-Tae-Eum-Pye-Gyeong
F Méridien des Poumons (P)
G Lungen Meridian (LU)
R Меридиан легких
V Phe-Kinh
L Cardinalis Pulmonalis Yin Maioris Manus (cP)
E Greater Yin, Large Yin, Arm Greater Yin, Lung Channel

X. Large intestine/Colon

P Intestinum Crassum Meridian (IC)
W-G Shou Yang Ming Ta Chang Ching (Li)
J Te no Yōmeidaichōkei
K Su-Yang-Myeong-De-Jang-Gyeong
F Méridien du Gros Intestin (GI)
G Dickdarm-Meridian (DI)
R Меридиан толстой кишки
V Kinh Dai-Truong
L Cardinalis Intestini Crassi Splendoris Yang Manus (cIC)
E Colon, Sunlight Yang, Sunshine Yang, Bright Yang, Yang Equilibrium, Middle Yang, Arm Yang Ming, Large Intestine Channel

XI. Stomach

P Ventriculus Meridian (V)
W-G Tsu Yang Ming Wei Ching (S)
J Ashi no Yōmeiikei
K Jog-Yang-Myeong-Wi-Gyeong
F Méridien de l'Estomac (E)
G Magen Meridian (M)
R Меридиан желудка
V Kinh Vi
L Cardinalis Stomachi Splendoris Yang Pedis (cS)
E Sunlight Yang, Bright Yang, Sunshine Yang, Yang Equilibrium Middle Yang, Leg Yang Ming, Stomach Channel

XII. Spleen/Pancreas

P Lien Pancreas Meridian (LP)
W-G Tsu Tai Yin Pi Ching (SP)
J Ashi no Taiinhikei
K Jog-Tae-Eum-Bi-Gyeong
F Méridien de la Rate-Pancreas (RP)
G Mirz-Pankreas-Meridian (MP)
R Меридиан селезенки
V Kinh Ty
L Cardinalis Lienalis Yin Maioris Pedis (cL)
E Pancreas, Greater Yin, Large Yin, Leg Greater Yin, Spleen Channel

---

P = Pinyin Chinese · W-G = Wade-Giles Chinese · J = Japanese
K = Korean · F = French · G = German · R = Russian
V = Vietnamese · L = Latin · E = English

	XIII. Conception Vessel	Worsley
	Ren Mai (CV)	Pinyin
Extra I	Jen Mo	Wade-Giles, French
	Jen Mei	Chancellor
	Ren Mo	F. Mann
	Im-Maeg-Gyeong	Korean
	Ninmyaku	Japanese
	Konzeptionsgefass, Jenn Mo	German
	Nham Mach	Vietnamese
	Передний срединный меридиан	Russian
	Front Midline Channel	Bensky & O'Connor
	Sinarteria Respondens	Latin

	XIV. Governor Vessel	Worsley
	Du Mai (GV)	Pinyin
Extra II	Tu Mo	Wade-Giles
	Tou Mo	French
	Tu Mei	Chancellor
	Du Mo	F. Mann
	Dog-Maeg-Gyeong	Korean
	Tokumyaku	Japanese
	Lenkergefass, Tou mo	German
	Doc Kinh	Vietnamese
	Задний срединный меридиан	Russian
	Backline Channel	Bensky & O'Connor
	Sinarteria Regens	Latin

Pinyin = Qi Jing
Wade Giles = chi-ching pa-mo
Korean & English = Eight extra meridians
French = méridiens curieux
Merveilleux vaisseaux
Méridiens particuliers
Méridiens irreguliers
Latin = Cardinales impares

Ns	K	P	W	M	L	
	Chung Maeg Penetrating Vessel	Chong Mai Vital Channel	Chong Mo Vessel of the Groin	Penetrating Vessel	Sinarteria Impedimentalis	
EIII.1	ST 30		ST 30	ST 30	ST 30	
EIII.2	KI 11	KI 11	KI 11	KI 11	KI 11	***Extra III***
EIII.3	KI 12	KI 12	KI 12	KI 12	KI 12	
EIII.4	KI 13	KI 13	KI 13	KI 13	KI 13	
EIII.5	KI 14	KI 14	KI 14	KI 14	KI 14	
EIII.6	KI 15	KI 15	KI 15	KI 15	KI 15	
EIII.7	KI 16	KI 16	KI 16	KI 16	KI 16	
EIII.8	KI 17	KI 17	KI 17	KI 17	KI 17	
EIII.9	KI 18	KI 18	KI 18	KI 18	KI 18	
EIII.10	KI 19	KI 19	KI 19	KI 19	KI 19	
EIII.11	KI 20	KI 20	KI 20	KI 20		
EIII.12	KI 21	KI 21	KI 21	KI 21	KI 21	
				CV 1	CV 1	
				CV 7		

Ns	K	P	W	M	L	
	Dae Maeg Girdle Vessel	Dai Mai Belt Channel	Dai Mo Vessel of the Waist	Girdle Vessel	Sinarteria Zonalis	
			LV 13	LV 13	LV 13	
EIV.1	GV 26	GV 26	GV 26	GV 26	GV 26	***Extra IV***
EIV.2	GV 27	GV 27	GV 27	GV 27	GV 27	
EIV.3	GV 28	GV 28	GV 28	GV 28	GV 28	

Ns = Numbered system • K = Korean • P = Pinyin Chinese
W = Worsley • M = Mann • L = Latin

	Ns	K	P	W	M	L
		Yang-Gyo-Maeg Yang Heel Vessel	Yang Chiao Mai Motility Channel of Yang	Yang Quiao Yang Vessel of the Ankle	Yang Heel Vessel	Sinarteria Ascendens Yang
Extra V	EV.1	BL 62	BL 62	BL 62	BL 62	BL 62
	EV.2	BL 61	BL 61	BL 61	BL 61	BL 61
	EV.3	BL 59	BL 59	BL 59	BL 59	BL 59
	EV.4	GL 38				
	EV.5	GB 29	GB 29		GB 29	GB 29
	EV.6	SI 10	SI 10	SI 10	SI 10	SI 10
	EV.7	LI 15	LI 15	LI 15	LI 15	LI 15
	EV.8	LI 16	LI 16	LI 16	LI 16	LI 16
	EV.9	ST 9			ST 7	
	EV.10	ST 4	ST 4	ST 4	ST 4	ST 4
	EV.11	ST 3	ST 3	ST 3	ST 6	ST 3
	EV.12	ST 1	ST 1	ST 1		ST 1
	EV.13	BL 1	BL 1	BL 1	BL 1	BL 1
	EV.14	GB 20		GB 20	GB 20	GB 20

Ns = Numbered system • K = Korean • P = Pinyin Chinese
W = Worsley • M = Mann • L = Latin

Ns	K	P	W	M	L
	Eum-Gyo-Maeg Eum Heel Vessel	Yin Chiao Mai Motility Channel of Yin	Yin Quiao Mo Yin Vessel of the Ankle	Yin Linking Vessel	Sinarteria Ascendens Yin
EVI.1	KI 2		KI 2		
EVI.2	KI 3			KI 3	KI 3
EVI.3	KI 6	KI 6	KI 6		KI 6
EVI.4	KI 8	KI 8	KI 8	KI 8	
EVI.5	ST 12				
EVI.6	ST 9				
EVI.7	BL 1	BL 1	BL 1	BL 1	BL 1

Extra VI

Ns = Numbered system • K = Korean • P = Pinyin Chinese
W = Worsley • M = Mann • L = Latin

	Ns	K	P	W	M	L
		Yang-Yu-Maeg Yang Linking Vessel	Yang Wei Mai Regulating Channel of Yang	Yang Wei Mo Vessel gathering the Yang	Yin Heel Vessel	Sinarteria Retinens Yang
	EVII.1	BL 63	BL 63		BL 63	BL 63
Extra VII	EVII.2	GB 35	GB 35	GB 35	GB 35	GB 35
	EVII.3	GB 29		GB 29		
	EVII.4	GB 24			GB 24	
	EVII.5	LI 14				LI 14
	EVII.6	TH 13		TH 13		TH 13
	EVII.7	SI 10	SI 10	SI 10	SI 10	
	EVII.8	TH 15	TH 15	TH 14	TH 15	TH 15
	EVII.9	GB 21	GB 21	GB 21	GB 21	GB 21
	EVII.10	ST 8	ST 8			
	EVII.11	GB 13	GB 13	GB 13	GB 13	GB 13
	EVII.12	GB 14	GB 14	GB 14	GB 14	GB 14
	EVII.13	GB 15	GB 15	GB 15	GB 15	GB 15
	EVII.14	GB 16	GB 16	GB 16	GB 16	GB 16
	EVII.15	GB 17	GB 17	GB 17	GB 17	GB 17
	EVII.16	GB 18	GB 18	GB 18	GB 18	GB 18
	EVII.17	GB 19	GB 19	GB 19	GB 19	GB 19
	EVII.18	GB 20	GB 20	GB 20		GB 20
	EVII.19	GV 16	GV 16			
			GV 15			LI 10

Ns = Numbered system • K = Korean • P = Pinyin Chinese
W = Worsley • M = Mann • L = Latin

Extra VIII

Ns	K	P	W	M	L
	Eum-Yu-Maeg Eum Linking Vessel	Yin Wei Mai Regulating Channel of Yin	Yin Wei Mo Vessel gathering the Yin	Yin Linking Vessel	Sinarteria Retinens Yin
EVIII.1	KI 9	KI 9		KI 9	KI 9
EVIII.2	SP 13	SP 13	SP 13	SP 13	SP 13
EVIII.3	SP 15	SP 15	SP 15	SP 15	SP 15
EVIII.4	SP 16	SP 16	SP 16	SP 16	SP 16
EVIII.5	LV 14	LV 14	LV 14	LV 14	LV 14
EVIII.6	CV 22	CV 22	CV 22	CV 22	CV 22
EVIII.7	CV 23	CV 23	CV 23	CV 23	CV 23
			SP 11	SP 12	

Ns = Numbered system • K = Korean • P = Pinyin Chinese
W = Worsley • M = Mann • L = Latin

12 INTERNAL MERIDIANS

These interconnect the primary meridians.

Internal pathways
Divergent channels
Collaterals
Piets

15 MERIDIANS WHICH CONNECT ENERGETIC SYSTEMS WITHIN THE SAME ELEMENT OR PHASE

Lo
Luo
Passage
Connecting
Junction

As adult bodies are proportionally the same the Chinese have utilized a unit defined as the size of the width of an individual's thumb, eye, or the distance between the distal first and second joints of the third finger as the measuring tool to determine the placement of acupuncture points.

A.U.M. = Acupuncture Unit of Measurement, by M. Austin

A.C.I. = Acupuncture Chinese Inch, by J.R. Worsley

Pounce = Inch, by W. W. Ping

Cun = Recent Chinese Texts

Unit = by J. O'Connor & D. Bensky

Osteological unit, osteo inch, by H.C. Lu

Cubic inch

SEVEN RADICALS

(SHEN, QI, YING, WEI, BLOOD, CHING-i, CHING/TZING)

SHEN (chen) guiding SPIRIT unconscious activities which resides in the HEART

PO (pro)
directs physical energies; chi, wei chi, blood, human senses, body movement, & voices. Related to FORM. Resides in the LUNG.

HUN (roun)
directs thinking, conscious and unconscious activity. Related to QI. Resides in the LIVER.

I (yi)
directs recollection. Resides in SPLEEN.

CHEN (zhi, tche)
directs process of will. Resides in the KIDNEY.

YUAN QI
(Source, yuann, congenital, inheritance, primordial, énergie originelle, ch'i nativum, essence, prenatal, genetic, original)

UTH

CHUNG QI
Derived from air
(Zong Qi, Zhong qi, Kong-qi, Dsong Qi,Da Qi, essential chi, ancestral energy, heavenly energy, Ta Tchi, Tien chi, ch'i caeleste, celestial qi).
Within lungs & heart.

MTH

KU QI
Derived from food and liquids
(Kou Qi, gu-qi, grain qi, Kou Tchi, ch'i, frumentarium, nutrient Qi).
Within stomach & spleen.

CHEN QI
(acquired chi, functional chi, Zhen Qi, Yuen Qi, general Qi, énergie essentielle acquise, ch'i merum, true energy, basic energy, genuine)
Material — Substance

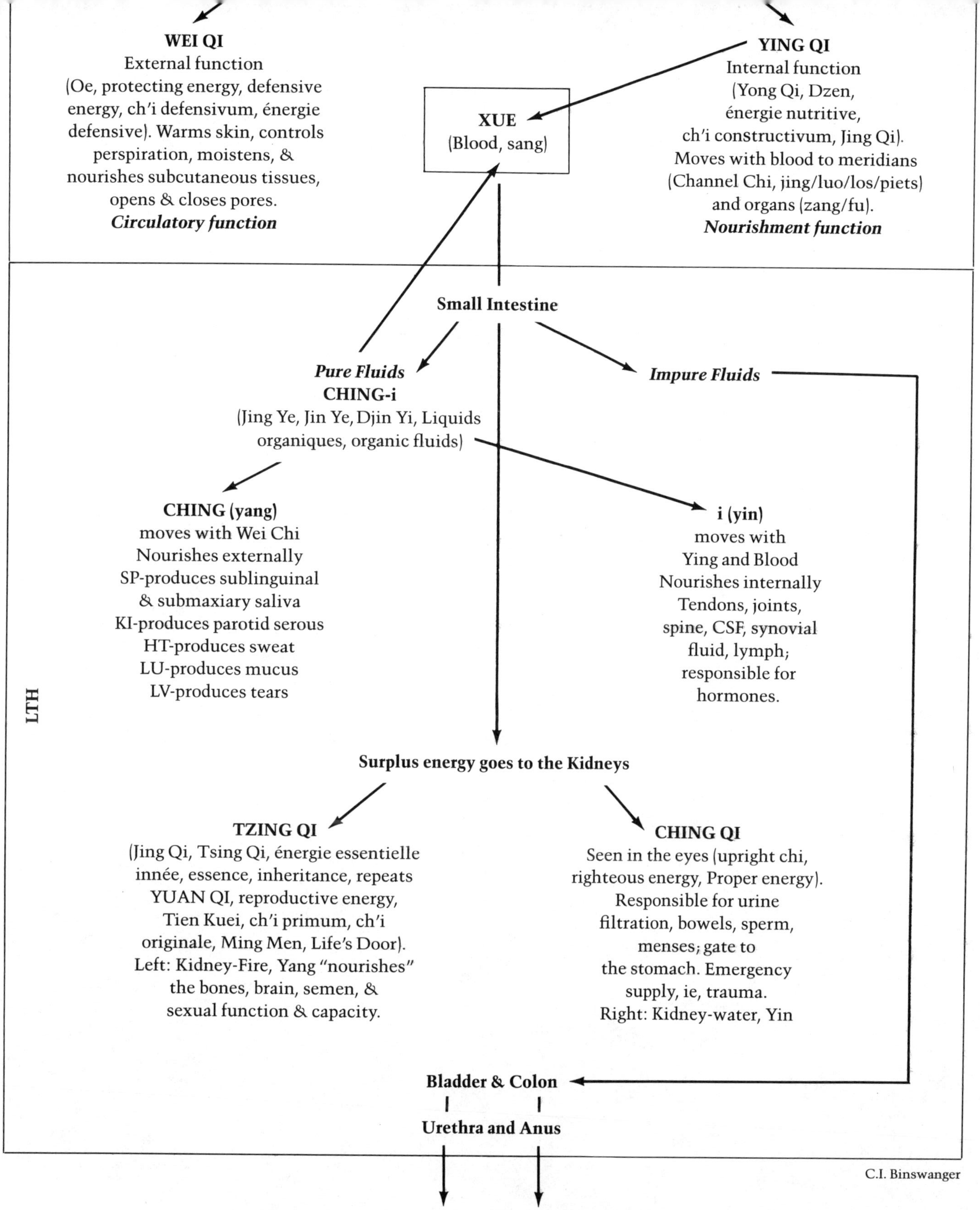

C.I. Binswanger

TITLE AND AUTHOR					
Five Shu Points An Outline of Chinese Medicine Academy of Traditional Chinese Medicine	Jing-Well	Yung-Spring	Shu-Stream	Jing-River	He-Sea
Five Shu Points Essentials of Chinese Acupuncture Traditional Chinese Medical Colleges; Beijing, Shanghai, Nanjing	Jing-Well	Rong-Spring	Shu Stream	Jing-River	He-Sea
Five Transporting Points Acupuncture, A Comprehensive Text O'Connor & Bensky	Well	Gushing	Transporting	Transversing	Uniting
Antique Points Acupuncture Therapeutic Pocket Book J.R. Worsley	Pt of Cheng Winter	Pt of Yung Spring	Pt of Yu Summer	Pt of Ching Late summer	PtHo Autumn
The Five Categories Acupuncture, The Ancient Chinese Art Felix Mann	Well emerging	Gushing flowing	Transporting pouring	Penetrating moving	Uniting entering
Su Antiques Semiologie et Therapeutique Nguyen Van Nghi & Mai Van Dong	Ting	Iong	Iu	King	Ho
Su Antiques Terrain et Pathologie en Acupuncture, Vol. II. Yves Requena	Ting	Yong ou Iong	Yu	King	Ho

CHINESE (Pinyin) Wang, Deshen, *Regional Working Group on the Standardization of Acupuncture Nomenclature*, Chinese Acupuncture & Moxibloxion, Vol 3, #4, 1983, and Vol 2, #6, 1982.

CHINESE (Pinyin) *Acupuncture Points Hanging Illustration Description Booklet*, Edited by: Hu Lion, Jin Shi-Ying, Jin Wan-Cheng. People's Health Publisher, New China Bookstores Beijing Distributor, 3rd printing, 2nd ed. Nov. 1983.

CHINESE (Wade-Giles) *Charts of Acupuncture Points and Meridians*, The Chinese Traditional Medical College of Shanghai & The Institute of Chinese Traditional Medicine of Shanghai, Pub: Shanghai Scientific & Technical Publishers, Shanghai, China, 1980.

JAPANESE *Names and Standard Location of Meridian Points*, Japanese Points Committee, 1976.

KOREAN *Standard Symbols of Meridians & Acupuncture Points*, Korean Oriental Medical Doctor's Association, Headquarters of W.C.A., 1975.

FRENCH Morant, Soulie de, *L'Acupuncture Chinoise*, Paris, 1939.

GERMAN Bachmann, Gerhard, *Leirfaden der Akupunktur*, Karl F. Haug Verlag, Ulm-Donau, 1961.

RUSSIAN Usova, M.K. & Morkhov, S.A., *Kratko rukovodstvo po ugloukalyvaniu i prizhiganiu*, Meditsina, 1974.

LATIN Porkert, Manfred, *The Theoretical Foundations of Chinese Medicine*, MIT Press, Cambridge, Mass., 1974.

ENGLISH

a) Lu, Henry C. *True Story of Chinese Acupuncture*, Vol. II, Academy of Oriental Heritage, Vancouver, 1976.

b) Ohashi, Wataru, Shiatsu Education Center of America, NYC.

c) Worsley, J.R., *The Meridians of Ch'i Energy: Point Reference Guide*, Centre of Traditional Acupuncture, Columbia, Md., 1976.

d) O'Connor, John, & Bensky, Dan, *Acupuncture, A Comprehensive Text*, Eastland Press, Chicago, 1981.

ADDITIONAL TITLES

Chamfrault., A., *Le Traité de la Médecine chinoise*, Angouleme, 1954.

de la Fuye, R., *Le Traité de Acupuncture chinoise*, Paris, 1955-6.

Karkow, O., *Akupunktur und International Nomenkuratur*, Deutsche Zeitschrift fur Akupunktur, Bd. III Ht. 5-6 S 36, 1954.

Lavier, J., *Théorie et pratique de l'Acupuncture et de Moxa*, 1960.

Lavier, J., *Points of Chinese Acupuncture*, Health Science Press, Rustington, Sussex, 1965.

Mann, Felix, *The Treatment of Disease by Acupuncture*, Wm. Heinemann, London, 1974.

Oteo, Francisco Méndez, Editor; *Fundeamentos de Acupunctura China*, Academia de Medicina Tradicional China, 3rd ed., Mexico 20. D.F., 1984.

Requena, Yves, *Terrain et Pathologie en Acupuncture*, Vol II , pp.635-7, Ed. Maline, Paris, 1982.

Tchao Ming-Te with *Intellectuelle des Sciences Sino-Internationales*, Pub-Tchao Ming-Te, Paris, 1967.